How to Dance

How to Dance

Second Edition

Formerly published as *Ballroom Dances*

Thomas E. Parson

PERENNIAL LIBRARY

Harper & Row, Publishers, New York
Cambridge, Philadelphia, San Francisco, Washington
London, Mexico City, São Paulo, Singapore, Sydney

This work was originally published by Barnes & Noble, Inc. under the title *Ballroom Dances*.

First PERENNIAL LIBRARY edition published 1986.

Library of Congress Cataloging-in-Publication Data

Parson, Thomas E.
How to dance.

"Perennial Library."
1. Ballroom dancing. I. Title.
GV1751.P28 1986 793.3'3 86-45134
ISBN 0-06-097052-9 (pbk.)

---

86 87 88 89 90 MPC 10 9 8 7 6 5 4 3 2 1

Preface

HISTORY reveals little of the origin of dancing except to substantiate the fact that the desire to dance is basic to the nature of man; otherwise it could not have survived and continued in use for century after century, from early biblical times to the present. There are allusions to dancing in the records of almost every nation, whether barbarian or civilized. Some mythological writers have stated that dancing was originally conceived and taught by Pollux and Castor to the Lacedaemonians; others have asserted that the credit should go to Minerva, who "after the defeat of the giants, danced for joy." In Scripture there is ample evidence that dancing formed a part of the religious ceremonies of the ancient Hebrews. Moses' triumph over the Egyptians was followed by singing and dancing (Exodus, 15:20). David, King of the Jews, danced before the Lord with all his might as he accompanied the ark (2 Samuel, 6:14). The Israelites danced at the inauguration of the Golden Calf (Exodus, 32:19). In the New Testament, dancing is mentioned in the parable of the Prodigal Son (Luke 15:29).

One of the first dances to be given a name was the Armed Dance, in which the dancers were "armed with sword, javelin and buckler." It was invented to "celebrate the victory of the gods, and the overthrow of the Titans." Grecian youths amused themselves with this dance during the siege of Troy.

Plato described the dances of the ancients thus:

1) Military dances, which tended to make the body robust, active, and well-disposed for all the exercises of war.

2) Domestic dances, which had for their object an innocent and agreeable relaxation and amusement.

3) Mediatorial dances, used in expiations and sacrifices.

The dances of Plato's time have undergone, through the years, changes peculiar to people of all nations and races. As one writer, Cellarius, put it more than a century ago, "The spirit of dancing prevails almost beyond imagination among people of every race, creed, and color. They have been observed to be easily affected by the sounds made by the drumming of sticks upon an empty cask, the noise made by blowing into reeds, the chanting of varied words of thought." (Could this have been a forerunner to our present-day bongo drums, clarinets, and folk and rock singing?)

Dancing eventually became the target of both bitter denunciation and genuine praise. Early theologians discussed its propriety and rendered the verdict: "As many paces as a man maketh in dancing, so many paces doth he make toward hell." On the other hand, it is written that Socrates, in his declining years took dancing lessons of "the beautiful Aspasia," and admonished his friends: "You laugh because I pretend to dance like young people, and think me ridiculous to wish for the benefits of exercise so necessary to the body and to the elegance of deportment."

In the twentieth century, we state emphatically that dancing is the effect of man's desire to move in harmony with the cadence produced by the sounds of musical instruments. And we emphasize, "They move easiest who have learned to dance!"

The author claims no personal credit for the invention or origin of any of the dances herein described; rather, he is deeply indebted to his colleages in the Dance Educators of America, Inc., for the mutual exchange of ideas over a long period of years, and in particular to Blossom Kramer, for her untiring aid in helping to define the intricacies of the Discotheque Dances. This book will be to some readers the sole means of acquiring a working knowledge of the fundamentals necessary to becoming fairly proficient in social and folk dances. For many others, in particular group leaders and teachers whose duties include serving as dance instructors, it may be a source of ideas and step patterns to supplement those they already use. In either case, it is hoped that the author's efforts will make easier and shorter the road to even more enjoyable participation in this most popular pastime.

Contents

How to Dance

TERMS AND ABBREVIATIONS

These terms and abbreviations are part of the standard terminology used by dance teachers throughout the country. They eliminate the need for lengthy word pictures in the lessons to follow.

Arch............Bring free foot to side of supporting foot, knee slightly flexed. No weight.

Ball-ch...........Ball-change. A combination of Press (bwd) and Step-in-Place. Two changes of weight.

Bwd.............Backward.

Close............Bring free foot to side of supporting foot and change weight.

Ch-Pos..........Challenge Position. Partners face each other about three feet apart with no hand hold.

Cl-Pos...........Closed Position. Also called "Waltz Position." Partners face each other or look over each other's right shoulder. Man's left, lady's right hands clasped. His right hand is placed firmly between her left shoulder blade and waist; her left hand rests lightly on his right shoulder.

Con-Pos.........Conversational Position. Partners are side-by-side facing LOD, lady at man's right. Lady's left hand rests on man's right shoulder, his right hand at her waist; his left, her right hands not clasped. Both move in same direction.

Cortez...........(*Tango*) Backward on man's left foot, forward on lady's right foot. Foot is flat on floor, with knee flexed to allow slight body sway. Free foot points to opposite direction.

Dip.............(*Fox-Trot*) Same as Cortez.

Ct(s)...........Count(s).

Diag. . . . . Diagonal(ly).
Draw. . . . . Same as Close, except that weight is not shifted. The next step is on the same foot.
Fwd. . . . . Forward.
L or LF. . . . . Left Foot.
LOD. . . . . Line of Direction or Line of Dance.
Lt. . . . . Left (directional).
Meas. . . . . Measure
OB-Pos. . . . . Open Break Position. Partners face each other and man holds lady's right hand in his left hand.
Point. . . . . Extend free foot to position indicated, with toe touching floor. No weight.
Press. . . . . Exert pressure to ball of foot to allow other foot to be raised and lowered in place. (See ball-ch.)
Prom-Pos. . . . . Promenade Position. Same as Con-Pos, but with man's left and lady's right hands clasped.
Q. . . . . Quick Step. Weight sustained for one beat.
R or RF. . . . . Right Foot.
Rock. . . . . Step forward or backward on foot indicated with a rocking motion. Free foot is extended in opposite direction in point position.
Rt. . . . . Right (directional).
S. . . . . Slow Step. Weight sustained for two beats.
SIP. . . . . Step-in-Place. Raise and lower foot without changing position.
Strike. . . . . Same as Arch.
Swd. . . . . Sideward.
Tap or Touch. . . . Extend free foot to position indicated, touch floor with ball of foot. No weight.
Wt. . . . . Weight.
X L or X R. . . . . . Cross in back or in front as indicated.
&. . . . . Expressed "and."

Dance Fundamentals

RELATION OF POSTURE TO DANCING

THE phrase "if you can walk you can dance" is too often taken in a literal sense. As a result of this, disappointment is experienced when it is discovered that the manner in which walking is practiced by some people does not resemble dancing even in its most elementary form. It may be correctly assumed, however, that a relation between the two does exist; that is, the feet are moved from one point on the floor to another in both processes. It is, then, a natural conclusion that a person who can walk will be able to learn to dance.

Many of the common faults in walking which are reflected in dancing can be attributed to poor posture, the result of improper distribution of weight together with the manner in which the weight is transferred from one foot to the other.

In many cases, poor posture is cultivated by a careless attitude toward personal appearance; the individual permits his shoulders to sag, stomach to protrude, knees to bend, feet to drag. In short, his body appears to be in a perpetual slump. A physical education teacher might say that such a person "looks tired, thinks tired, walks tired!" He may admonish him to "look tall, think tall, walk tall!" The dance teacher will be heard adding the advice to "dance tall!"

A point well worth remembering is that good posture is absolutely essential to good dancing.

POSTURE CORRECTION

The first step in correcting poor posture is to learn how to *take a load off the feet.* Let's try it.

1. Stand in front of a mirror with your feet flat on the floor. Keep your heels together, the balls of your feet about four inches apart.

2. Now *stand tired:* let your body sag, your stomach protrude, your knees bend slightly. This will shorten your normal height about three inches.

3. At this point try swinging your right leg forward and backward. Your foot will drag heavily as it is moved to-and-fro.

4. Now start to *think tall!* From your ankles upward through your knees, thighs, and body, make yourself four inches taller.

5. Let your weight gradually shift forward onto the forepart of your feet. The heels remain touching the floor but with no weight on them.

6. Now raise your arms so that the upper arms are horizontal, the forearms vertical, and the palms forward.

7. Pretend that you are being raised to the ceiling from the top of your head. (Do not rise on your toes.)

8. Now swing your right leg forward and backward. Note that this time the foot does not drag.

9. Let your body sag downward. Now repeat the exercise and start swinging the leg as the body gains height.

Practiced diligently, this exercise will help you to THINK TALL . . . LOOK TALL . . . WALK TALL . . . AND DANCE TALL!

THE PROGRESSIVE

Forward Movement

Now start walking slowly forward. Place the left foot —*heel down first*—on a direct line in front of the right foot. Do not permit the body to sag as the weight is transferred. Now place the right foot—*heel down first*—on a direct line in front of the left foot. Keep the weight up! Keep on walking, very slowly, with weight up and chin out. Soon a swinging motion from the hips downward will be noticed. Remember, though, to walk—save the dancing for later. Remember, too, that each foot is placed directly in front of the other.

The object of this exercise is an unbroken flow of motion as the weight is shifted from one foot to the other. Practice this phase diligently.

Now the actual dance movement can be started. The *ball* of foot, instead of heel, is first to make contact with the floor. No other change is made in stance or stride! As before, each foot is placed directly in front of the other —this time with ball of foot down first. As the weight is received, push the foot forward just a few inches before a complete transfer is made. *Do not rise on toes*. Practice this phase diligently.

Backward Movement

Start with the right foot and walk slowly backward. Place the right foot on a direct line in back of the left. The inside of the big toe is first to feel the weight, which is then released to the ball of the foot. Now place the left foot on a direct line in back of the right, and so on, very slowly. Keep the chin up!

Keep the knees *straight but not stiff* as the weight is shifted. Do not permit the body to sag as weight is transferred. Practice with arms in same position as described for the forward movement.

Jointly referred to as the "progressive," the forward and backward movements will develop poise, balance, and graceful carriage (posture)—the essentials to *improved* walking or dancing. It is necessary, then, that the progressive movements be practiced at every opportunity.

THE SIDEWARD-CLOSE MOVEMENT

When the progressive movements have been developed to a point where the weight is carried upward to prevent slouching, the "sideward-close" is easily accomplished. Try it. Stand with heels and toes together. Raise the left heel, extend the left foot about twelve inches to the left side, on a line parallel with the right foot, and shift the weight to the left; now draw the right foot against the left and shift the weight to the right. Do this several times; then start with the right foot and do the sideward-close to the right.

Note particularly that the sideward-close is made up of two changes of weight—on the *sideward* movement and on the *closing* movement. Always remember this when combining the progressive and the sideward-close to create combinations for the Fox-Trot and other ballroom dances.

COMBINING THE PROGRESSIVE AND SIDEWARD-CLOSE

Taken singly, the progressive and the sideward-close become with practice simple operations; an attempt at combining the two can, however, create problems to be solved only by a thorough understanding of the basic principles of each, together with the close relation of one to the other.

For example, you have found in practice that the progressive movement is accomplished by placing one foot directly in front (or in back) of the other, by transferring the weight to that foot, and by following immediately with the other foot in the same direction. You have found, too, that the sideward-close is the result of moving one foot sideward (parallel with the other), transferring the weight to that foot, and immediately drawing the other alongside the first *with another transfer of weight!*

A combination well suited for practice, and containing all the elements of the foregoing, follows:

a) Stand with heels and toes together, arms raised;

b) start with left foot, take three steps forward on left, right, left, and end with weight on left;

c) with a continuous motion, draw the right foot forward until the ball of right is at side of and touching the heel of left, then move sideward on and transfer weight to rıght foot;

d) close left against right and shift weight to left;

e) start with right foot, take three backward steps on right, left, right, and end with weight on right;

f) with a continuous motion, draw the left foot backward until the heel of left is at side of and touching the fore part of right, then move sideward on and transfer weight to left foot;

g) close right against left and shift weight to right. *Start with left foot and repeat over and over.*

Abbreviated, this combination would be described as:

Fwd L-R-L—swd-close R-L
Bwd R-L-R—swd-close L-R.

SELF-ANALYZATION AND CORRECTION

Most of the difficulties encountered in effecting a combination of the progressive and sideward-close can be attributed (1) to a misunderstanding of the principles involving each, or (2) to a lack of ability heightened by failure to practice the application of these principles. In either case, there may be developed any of these three common faults:

1. Failure to move on a direct line forward (or backward), thus causing the feet to spread.
2. Failure to commence the sideward-close with a definite sideward movement, thus creating in many instances a duplication of the incorrect movement in fault 1.
3. Failure to shift the weight to the foot making the closing step in the sideward-close, which causes a start on the wrong foot.

These are but minor difficulties, to be overcome through a review and *closer* application of the basic principles of the progressive and sideward-close.

APPLICATION OF TIMING EFFECT

In some people there exists a natural inclination to respond with perfect timing to music played in any rhythm or tempo; in others the ability to keep time must be developed.

Dance music is played in even cadence, with a steady recurrence of certain beats to guide the dancer in both speed of movement and in determining the type of music being played—i.e., Waltz, Fox-Trot, Tango, Samba, etc.

The foregoing combination of the progressive and sideward-close is easily adapted to music played in 4/4, or Fox-Trot, time. Before proceeding, however, there must be established the difference between the meaning of (1) the musical count and (2) the dance count.

The *musical* count would represent the number and sequence of beats to the measure; for instance, 4/4 time denotes four beats (or musical counts) to the measure. Since a transfer of weight (or step) is not intended for each successive beat in Fox-Trot music, the *dance* count would denote the sequence of steps and whether the weight should be sustained on each succeeding transfer for two beats or for one, with these resultant expressions being used:

Slow Step (S): on which the weight is sustained for two beats, and

Quick Step (Q): on which the weight is sustained for one beat.

The application of Fox-Trot timing to the now familiar combination of progressive and sideward-close should provide a basis on which can be developed a sound working knowledge of the essentials necessary to become a good dancer.

Measure	Musical Count	Dance Count	Dance Movement	Time
1	1–2	1	Forward Left........	S
	3–4	2	Forward Right.......	S
2	1–2	3	Forward Left........	S
	3	4	Sideward Right......	Q
	4	and	Close Left to Right....	Q
3	1–2	5	Backward Right.....	S
	3–4	6	Backward Left.......	S
4	1–2	7	Backward Right.....	S
	3	8	Sideward Left........	Q
	4	and	Close Right to Left...	Q
			Repeat over and over from 1st count.	

THE SIMPLE TURNS

In establishing the basic approach to the simple turns, a single progressive combined with a sideward-close, reversed and repeated, is used. With their respective timing effects applied, this approach is standard for the Fox-Trot, Waltz, Tango, Samba, and Rumba.

It is advisable to develop the "feel" of the turning sequences before making an attempt at turning. For the left turn the sequence would be:

Fwd L—Swd-close R-L
Bwd R—Swd-close L-R

For the right turn the sequence is:

Fwd R—Swd-close L-R
Bwd L—Swd-close R-L

Once the feel of the approach to the turns has been developed, it is a simple matter to extend the movements into the desired turns. The accompanying diagrams show the approximate positions of the feet, together with the timing effect for the Fox-Trot. Note that perfect quarter-turns can be made on each turning sequence. The four walls of the room can be used as a guide in gauging the depth of the turns.

Left Turn (Fox-Trot Timing)

COUNT		TIME
1	Fwd L, turn to face center....	S
2-&	Swd-close R-L...	Q-Q
3	Bwd R, turn to face opposite LOD.........	S
4-&	Swd-close L-R...	Q-Q

Repeat to end facing LOD.

Figure 1

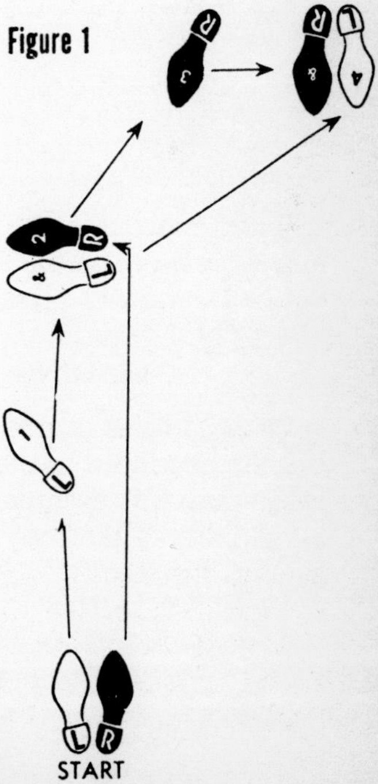

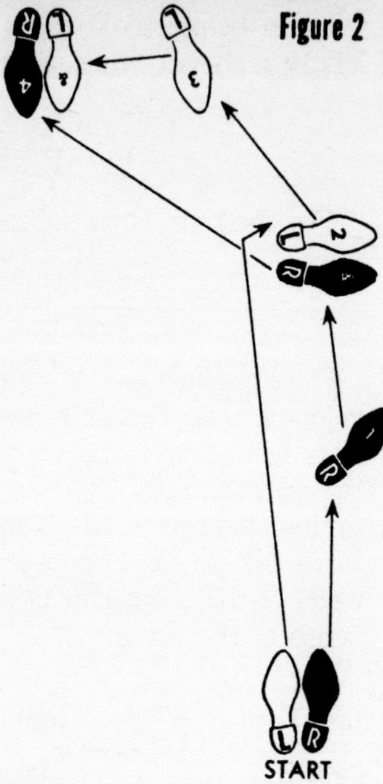

Figure 2

Right Turn (Fox-Trot Timing)

COUNT		TIME
1	Fwd R, turn to face wall	S
2-&	Swd-close L-R . . .	Q-Q
3	Bwd L, turn to face opposite LOD	S
4-&	Swd-close R-L . . .	Q-Q
	Repeat to end facing LOD.	

When practicing the turns with a partner, the lady moves *backward* on the R as the gentleman moves *forward* on the L, and vice versa.

LEADING AND FOLLOWING

In the process of mastering the simple basic technique there is developed in the dancer a co-ordination of movement that will eventually result in immediate response by all parts of the body to the impulses set up at the beginning of a step.

The man's lead would be described as "weak" if his body or his right arm should respond slowly to a forward, or to a turning, movement of the foot. And if his partner should continue with another backward step when he attempts a sideward-close he might again be blamed; but this might indicate, on the other hand, that the lady does not respond with sufficient ease to his lead.

It is obvious, then, that efficiency in both leading and following is to be measured in accordance with the individual's ability to consistently apply the aforementioned principles. It is also obvious that to effect a "strong" lead on his partner the man need not grasp her around the waist with a wrestler's hold.

A comfortable position having been taken by both partners, one in which both can move freely, the force necessary to propel the man's feet into predetermined positions will set up reactions throughout the body that will impel his partner to do the counterpart of his movement—*provided she is moving properly.*

The outward elements of leading and following can be summed up briefly. Both partners assume natural, comfortable positions. The man's elbows should be raised away from the body to an angle of at least forty-five degrees, or to a horizontal position. His right hand is placed at an advantageous spot between the lady's shoulders and waistline.

The lady's left arm should follow the line of the man's right arm, her left hand resting lightly on his right shoulder. *She must at all times carry her own weight.*

Both should retain a position in which each may look over the other's right shoulder. His left and her right hand may or may not be clasped, according to the style of dancing adopted at various times.

But above everything else—and to the exclusion of one or more of these generally-accepted rules—a natural attitude based on the principles already stressed should be assumed by both partners. Ballroom dancing is meant to be thoroughly enjoyed, and the pleasure derived from dancing with one partner as compared with another depends largely on the individual's knack of making his or her dancing conform to the laws of natural movement.

LINE OF DIRECTION

The counterclockwise course maintained in making progress around the dance floor is referred to as "Line of Direction" or "Line of Dance" (LOD).

When moving forward to LOD, the center of the room is at the man's left, the wall at his right; the lady, in moving backward to LOD, would have the center of the room at her right, the wall at her left.

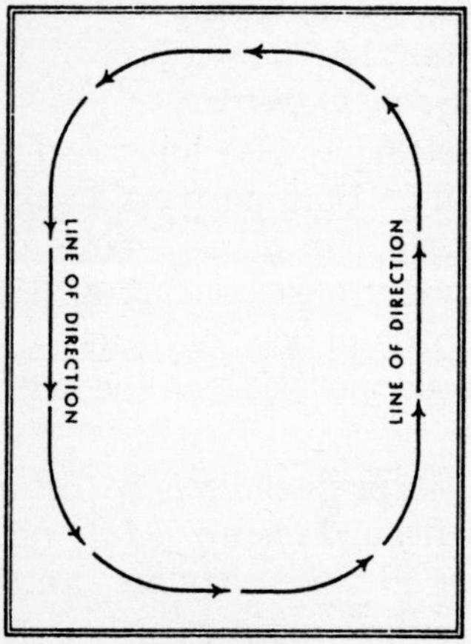

Figure 3

The necessity of adhering to the traffic rules of the dance floor should be obvious: it prevents unnecessary collisions and the confusion that would result if dancers were permitted to make progress in all directions.

The Fox-Trot

For several decades prior to 1914, many dances—the Polka, the Schottische, the Galop, the Mazurka, the Turkey Trot, the Bunny Hug, the Grizzly Bear, the One-Step, and the Two-Step (the two latter made danceable and popular by Vernon and Irene Castle)—vied for popularity in America. The music for all of these dances was bouncy and over-accented; the dancing followed suit. Bandleader Harry Fox, then playing at the old Amsterdam Roof Garden in New York City, tried out a few numbers with less bounce and more smoothness. Dancers responded by combining the One-Step and the Two-Step, and thus the Fox-Trot was born.

In the years that followed, many variations of the Fox-Trot became overnight sensations. In the early 1920's there was the Charleston; then came the Lindbergh Hop which evolved into the sensational Lindy, which still has its followers. The Shag was popular for a couple years. All these variations and many more were the result of varied accentuations of music written in 4/4 time, and were popularized by dancers gifted with the ability to express themselves to the music being played.

One of the reasons for the Fox-Trot's wide appeal among less gifted dancers is that the musical framework is not always in multiples of four, eight, or sixteen beats. As a consequence it is not a rhythm dance as the term is applied to the Charleston, the Cha-Cha, the Polka, or even the Waltz.

Figure 4

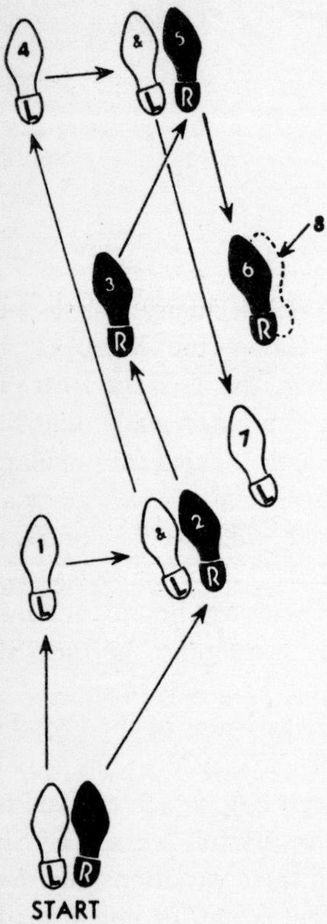

FIRST COMBINATION

Man's Part

COUNT		TIME
1	Fwd L..........	S
2-&	Swd-close R-L...	Q-Q
3	Fwd R.........	S
4	Fwd L..........	S
5-&	Swd-close R-L...	Q-Q
6	Bwd R.........	S
7	Dip bwd L......	S
8	Fwd R.........	S

Repeat from 1st count.

Figure 5

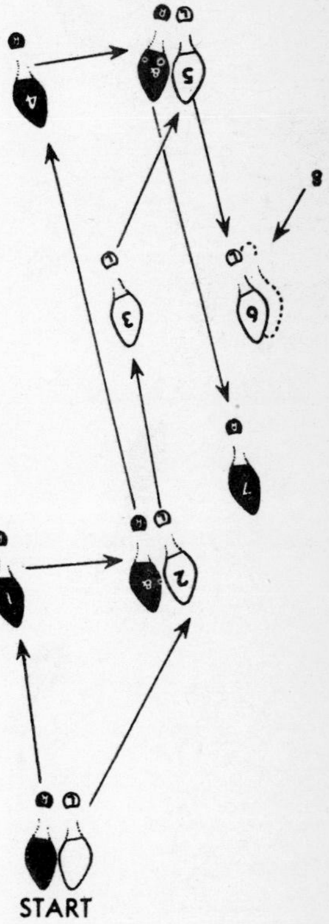

FIRST COMBINATION

Lady's Part

COUNT		TIME
1	Bwd R..........	S
2-&	Swd-close L-R...	Q-Q
3	Bwd L..........	S
4	Bwd R..........	S
5-&	Swd-close L-R...	Q-Q
6	Fwd L..........	S
7	Dip fwd R......	S
8	Bwd L..........	S

Repeat from 1st count.

Figure 6

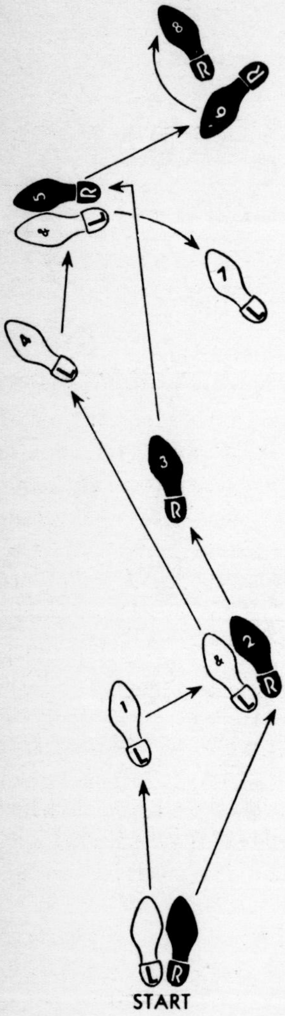

SECOND COMBINATION

Man's Part

Count		Time
1	Fwd L..........	S
2-&	Swd-close R-L...	Q-Q
3	Fwd R.........	S
4	Fwd L, turn to face center....	S
5-&	Swd-close R-L...	Q-Q
6	Bwd R.........	S
7	Dip bwd L, turn to LOD.......	S
8	Fwd R to face LOD.........	S

Repeat from 1st count or combine with previous combination.

Figure 7

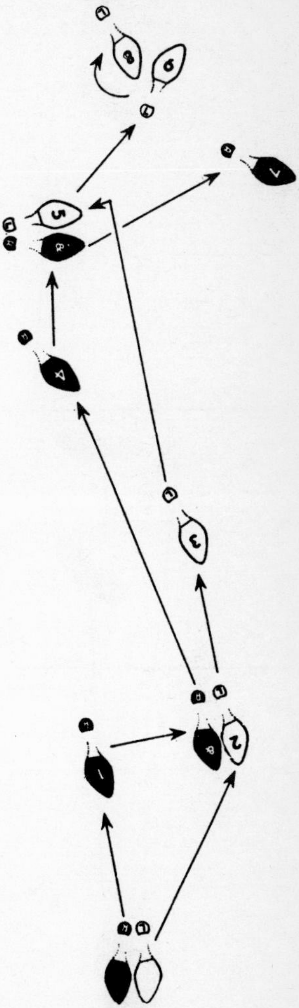

SECOND COMBINATION

Lady's Part

COUNT		TIME
1	Bwd R.	S
2-&	Swd-close L-R. . .	Q-Q
3	Bwd L.	S
4	Bwd R, turn to face wall	S
5-&	Swd-close L-R. . .	Q-Q
6	Fwd L.	S
7	Dip fwd R, turn to face opposite LOD	S
8	Bwd L to LOD. . .	S

Repeat from 1st count or combine with previous combination.

Figure 8

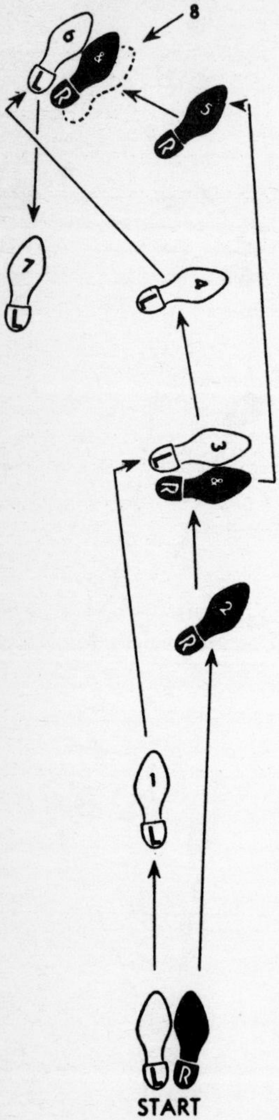

THIRD COMBINATION

Man's Part

COUNT		TIME
1	Fwd L..........	S
2	Fwd R, turn to face wall......	S
3-&	Swd-close L-R...	Q-Q
4	Swd L, to LOD..	S
5	Cross R between self and partner	S
6-&	Swd-close L-R, turn to LOD...	Q-Q
7	Dip bwd L......	S
8	Fwd R to face LOD.........	S

Repeat from 1st count.

Figure 9

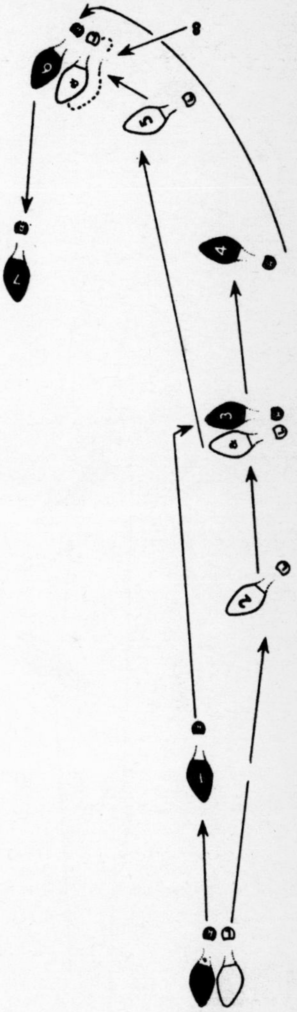

THIRD COMBINATION

Lady's Part

COUNT		TIME
1	Bwd R.........	S
2	Bwd L, turn to face center....	S
3-&	Swd-close R-L...	Q-Q
4	Swd R, to LOD..	S
5	Cross L between self and partner	S
6-&	Swd-close R-L, turn to opposite LOD.........	Q-Q
7	Dip fwd R.......	S
8	Bwd L to face opposite LOD....	S

Repeat from 1st count.

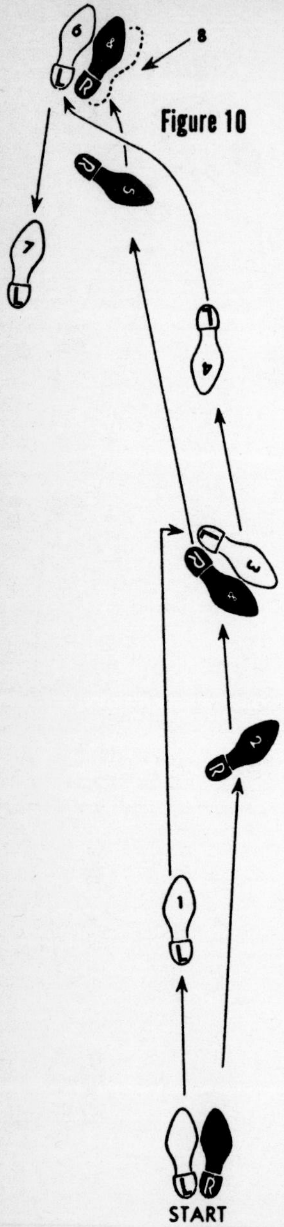

Figure 10

FOURTH COMBINATION

Man's Part

COUNT		TIME
1	Fwd L..........	S
2	Fwd R, turn to face wall......	S
3-&	Swd-close L-R, end facing opposite LOD....	Q-Q
4	Bwd L, opposite LOD.........	S
5	Bwd R, turn to face wall......	S
6-&	Swd-close L-R, end facing LOD	Q-Q
7	Dip bwd L......	S
8	Fwd R..........	S

Repeat from 1st count.

FOURTH COMBINATION

Lady's Part

COUNT		TIME
1	Bwd R..........	S
2	Bwd L, turn to face center....	S
3-&	Swd-close R-L, end facing LOD	Q-Q
4	Fwd R, to LOD..	S
5	Fwd L, turn to face center....	S
6-&	Swd-close R-L, end facing opposite LOD....	Q-Q
7	Dip fwd R.......	S
8	Bwd L..........	S

Repeat from 1st count.

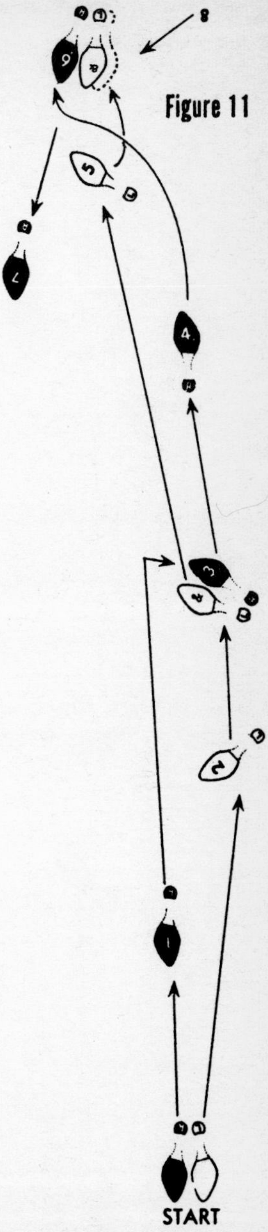

Figure 11

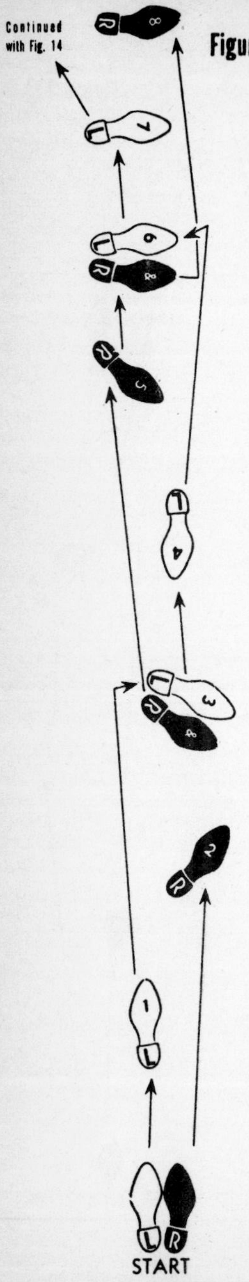

Figure 12

FIFTH COMBINATION

Man's Part

COUNT		TIME
1	Fwd L..........	S
2	Fwd R, turn to face wall......	S
3-&	Swd-close L-R, end facing opposite LOD...	Q-Q
4	Bwd L to LOD...	S
5	Bwd R, turn to face wall......	S
6-&	Swd-close L-R, end facing wall.	Q-Q
7	Swd L, to LOD..	S
8	Cross R between self and partner	S

Continue with 6th combination.

Figure 13

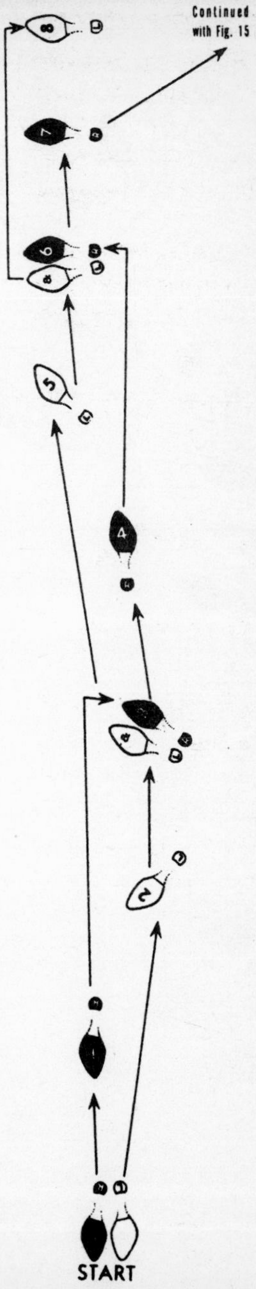

FIFTH COMBINATION

Lady's Part

COUNT		TIME
1	Bwd R..........	S
2	Bwd L, turn to face center....	S
3-&	Swd-close R-L, end facing LOD	Q-Q
4	Fwd R to LOD..	S
5	Fwd L, turn to face center....	S
6-&	Swd-close R-L, end facing center...........	Q-Q
7	Swd R to LOD...	S
8	Cross L between self and partner	S

Continue with 6th combination.

Figure 14

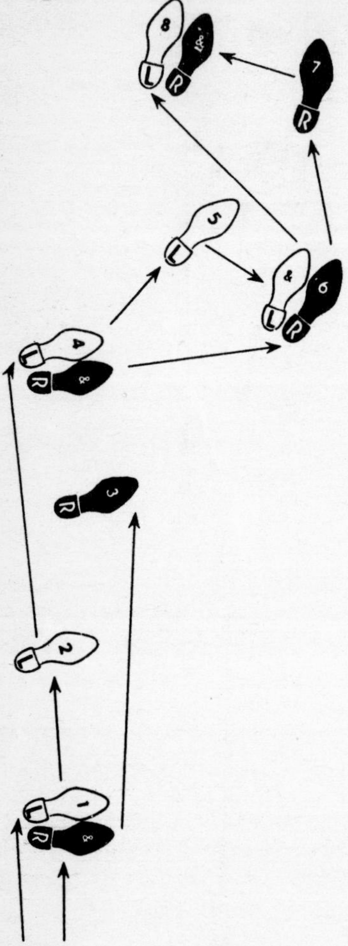

Continued from Fig. 12

SIXTH COMBINATION

Man's Part

COUNT		TIME
	Start facing wall:	
1-&	Swd-close L-R to LOD.......	Q-Q
2	Swd L..........	S
3	Cross R between self and partner	S
4-&	Swd-close L-R...	Q-Q
5	Fwd L to wall....	S
6-&	Swd-close R-L...	Q-Q
7	Cross R between self and partner	S
8-&	Swd-close L-R, end facing LOD	Q-Q

Repeat from 1st count of previous combination.

Figure 15

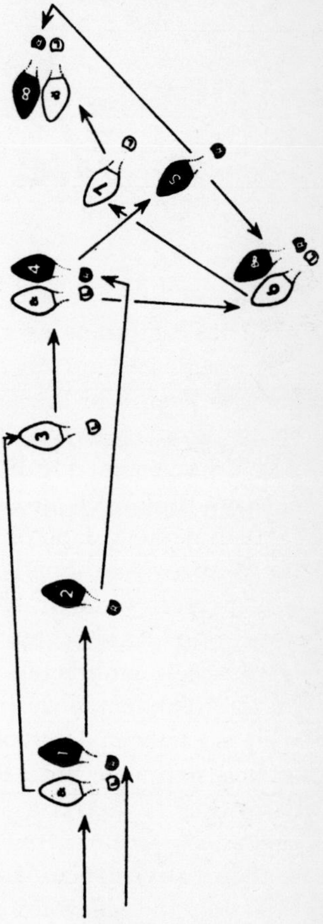

Continued

SIXTH COMBINATION

Lady's Part

Count		Time
	Start facing center:	
1-&	Swd-close R-L to LOD.......	Q-Q
2	Swd R..........	S
3	Cross L between self and partner	S
4-&	Swd-close R-L...	Q-Q
5	Bwd R to wall...	S
6-&	Swd-close L-R...	Q-Q
7	Cross L between self and partner	S
8-&	Swd-close R-L, end facing opposite LOD....	Q-Q

Repeat from 1st count of previous combination.

The Waltz

Some historians ascribe to the claim that the Waltz originated in Italy as La Volta and from there spread to France to become the Valse à trois temps. Others credit Germany as the source, pointing out that the Waltz was a movement ideally adaptable to the timing of the German tune "Ach du Lieber Augustin," first heard about 1770. But most dance historians agree that the home of the Waltz was originally Bavaria.

E. Ferrero wrote in 1847 that the Waltz originally consisted of a "leaping step forward and a leaping step backward, each embracing one measure (three beats) of music." The tempo was in excess of sixty bars per minute, so it is easily understood why the sideward step and the closing step were not used by the Bavarian peasants who, according to Ferrero, "without removing their wooden shoes, took time out from their labors in the fields to indulge in their native dance." Later the Waltz was modernized by injecting the sideward step on the second beat and the closing step on the third beat of the measure.

Basically the Waltz today is the same as it was in the eighteenth and nineteenth centuries. The principle of accenting the step corresponding to the first beat of the measure of music has remained intact. Written in 3/4 time, Waltz music presents a problem not found in 2/4 or 4/4 time; there is an odd number of beats on which the sound and step pattern is constructed. As a result, too many dancers employ a pattern in which the closing step is made on the wrong beat of the measure. Executed properly, the closing step in the Waltz is made on the third or sixth step in the pattern, each corresponding with the third beat of the measure: forward (or backward), sideward, *close.*

SOUND AND BASIC STEP PATTERN

Listen to any old-time Waltz: "The Blue Danube," "Ach du lieber Augustin," or to one in slower tempo. In each will be heard a definite accent on the first beat of the measure, followed by two softer beats: ONE-two-three, ONE-two- three. The weight is sustained on each step for the same length of time, hence slow and quick steps are not involved as in other dances. Also, the dance count and the music count are the same, thus eliminating the need for the "and" count as used in 2/4 and4/4 timing.

To simplify teaching the Waltz, the three changes of weight made in each measure are together known as the *Waltz Step;* when alternated forward and backward, two Waltz Steps become the *Box-Step.* Dancing forward (man's part) or backward (lady's part) without alternating creates the *Progressive.* Since the Box-Step is the basis for the Left and Right Turns, this pattern should be diligently practiced.

The Left Box (2 measures)

Man:	Fwd L	Swd R	Cl L	Bwd R	Swd L	Cl R
	1	2	3	4	5	6
Lady:	Bwd R	Swd L	Cl R	Fwd L	Swd R	Cl L

The Right Box (2 measures)

Alternate: man starts Bwd L, lady Fwd R.

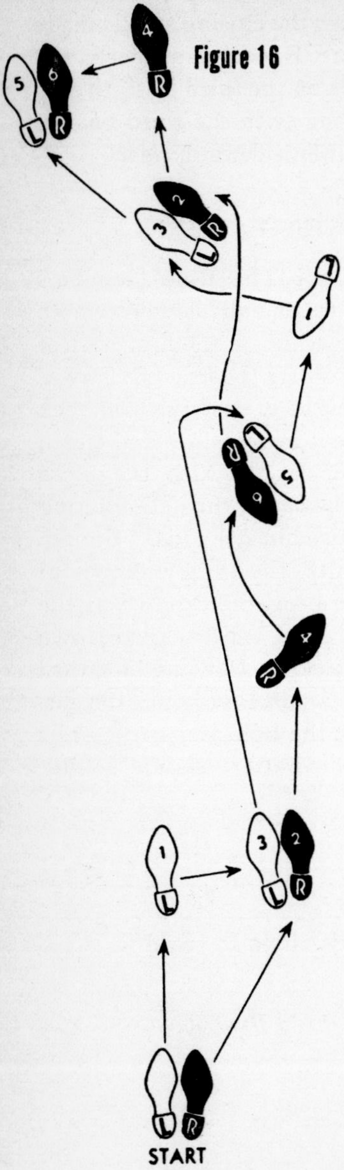

Figure 16

FIRST COMBINATION

Man's Part—The Right Turn

COUNT

Count	Step	
1	Fwd L	
2	Swd R	
3	Close L	
4	Fwd R	*Turn Rt. to face wall, end facing opposite LOD.*
5	Swd L	
6	Close R	
1	Bwd L	*Turn Rt. to face center, end facing LOD.*
2	Swd R	
3	Close L	
4	Fwd R	
5	Swd L	
6	Close R	

FIRST COMBINATION

Lady's Part—The Right Turn

COUNT		
1	Bwd R	
2	Swd L	
3	Close R	
4	Bwd L	*Turn Rt. to face center, end facing LOD.*
5	Swd R	
6	Close L	
1	Fwd R	*Turn Rt. to face wall, end facing opposite LOD.*
2	Swd L	
3	Close R	
4	Bwd L	
5	Swd R	
6	Close L	

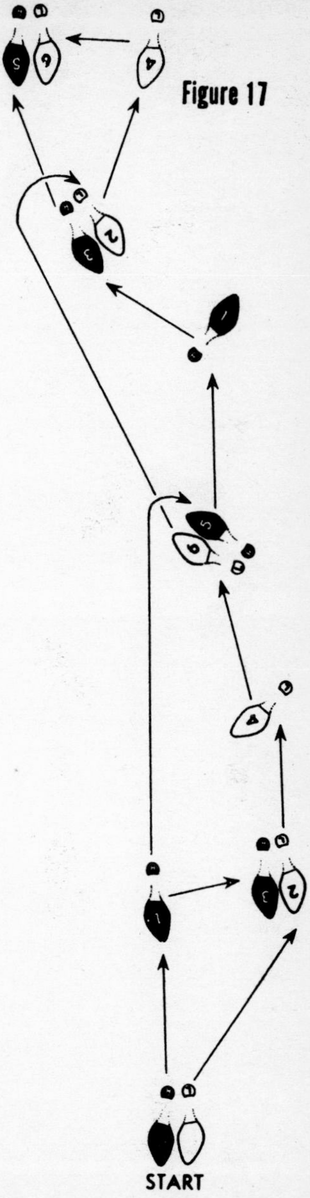

Figure 17

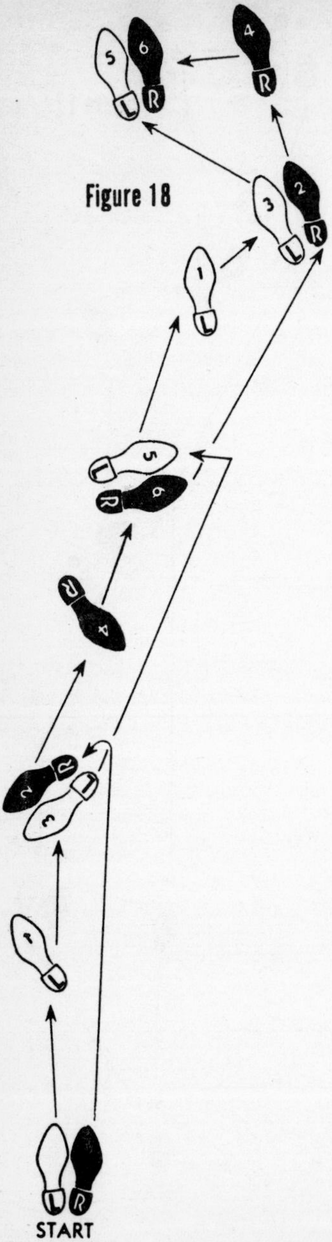

Figure 18

SECOND COMBINATION

Man's Part—The Left Turn

COUNT

Count	Step	
1	Fwd L	*Turn Lt. to face center, end facing opposite LOD.*
2	Swd R	
3	Close L	
4	Bwd R	*Turn Lt. to face wall.*
5	Swd L	
6	Close R	
1	Fwd L	*Turn Lt. to end facing LOD.*
2	Swd R	
3	Close L	
4	Fwd R	
5	Swd L	
6	Close R	

SECOND COMBINATION

Lady's Part—The Left Turn

COUNT		
1	Bwd R	*Turn Lt. to face wall, end facing LOD.*
2	Swd L	
3	Close R	
4	Fwd L	*Turn Lt. to face center.*
5	Swd R	
6	Close L	
1	Bwd R	*Turn Lt. to end facing opposite LOD.*
2	Swd L	
3	Close R	
4	Bwd L	
5	Swd R	
6	Close L	

Figure 19

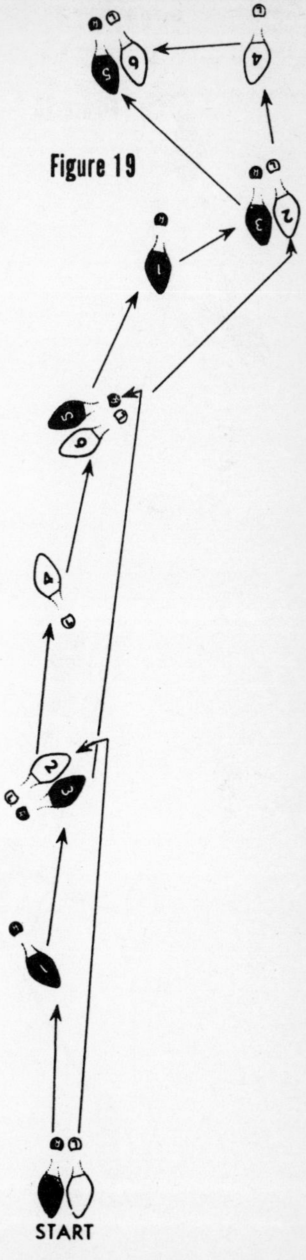

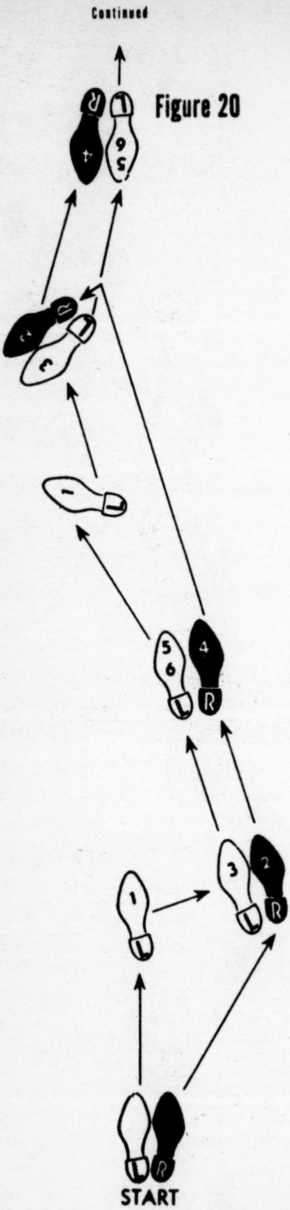

Figure 20

THIRD COMBINATION

Man's Part—The Hesitation

COUNT

1 Fwd L

2 Swd R

3 Close L

4 Fwd R

5–6 Draw L to R, no weight on L

1	Fwd L	*Turn Lt. to face center, end facing opposite LOD.*
2	Swd R	
3	Close L	

4 Bwd R to LOD

5–6 Draw L to R, no weight on L

Continue with 4th combination.

THIRD COMBINATION

Lady's Part—The Hesitation

COUNT

1 Bwd R

2 Swd L

3 Close R

4 Bwd L

5–6 Draw R to L, no weight on R

1 Bwd R
2 Swd L
3 Close R
} *Turn Lt. to face wall, end facing LOD.*

4 Fwd L to LOD

5–6 Draw R to L, no weight on R

Continue with 4th combination.

Figure 21

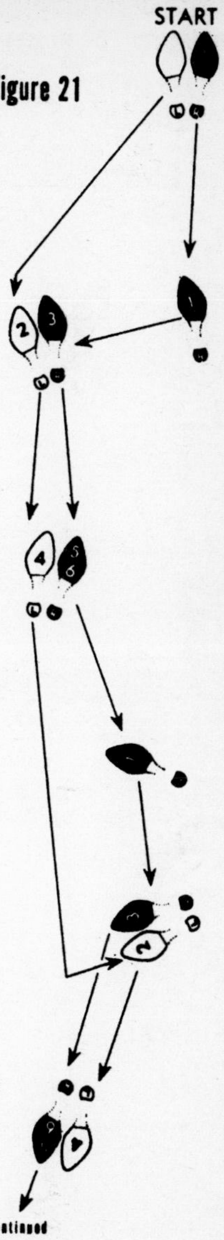

FOURTH COMBINATION

Figure 22

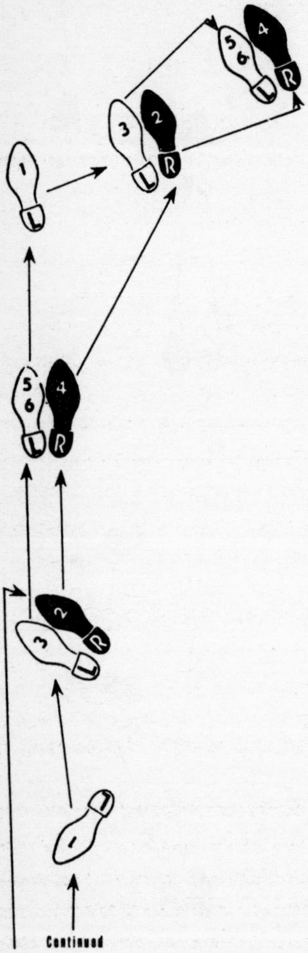

Man's Part—The Hesitation

COUNT

Start facing opposite LOD:

1 Bwd L
2 Swd R
3 Close L
(1–3: Turn Rt. to face center end facing LOD.)

4 Fwd R to LOD

5–6 Draw L to R, no weight on L

1 Fwd L

2 Swd R

3 Close L

4 Swd R to wall

5–6 Draw L to R, no weight on L

Repeat from beginning of 3rd combination.

FOURTH COMBINATION

Lady's Part—The Hesitation

Figure 23

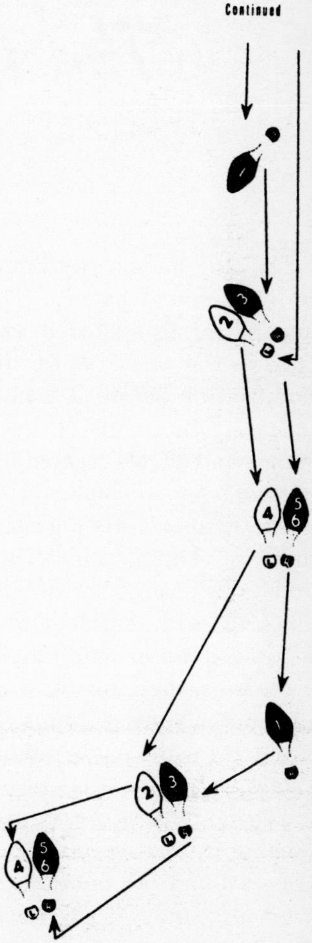

COUNT

Start facing LOD:

1 Fwd R
2 Swd L
3 Close R
} *Turn Rt. to face wall, end facing opposite LOD.*

4 Bwd L to LOD

5–6 Draw R to L, no weight on R

1 Bwd R

2 Swd L

3 Close R

4 Swd L to wall

5–6 Draw R to L, no weight on R

Repeat from beginning of 3rd combination.

The Rumba

The Rumba is a rhythm dance, a constant repetition of the basic sound pattern. This, together with its simplified step patterns, makes it easy to learn. Introduced from Cuba in the early 1930's, the Rumba needed considerable modification before it was finally accepted as a ballroom dance. Its music, in 4/4 time, was a mixture of ear-pleasing sounds and effects created by Latin American instruments: *maracas, claves, bongo* and *conga drums, cenceros, guiros.*

The Rumba's distinguishing feature is the style of the body movement which is applied to an exceptionally simple pattern of steps. This movement is not wholly in character with that developed in the Waltz, Fox-Trot, and Tango; it can be said that it is typically Latin American. It remains, then, for the dancer to concentrate on mastering Rumba style, without which even a perfect application of sound to step pattern would resemble too closely a Fox-Trot.

The Rumba is a non-progressive dance, with couples dancing in relatively small areas rather than making progress around the floor. As a consequence, one of the first items of study is to learn to take small steps and to *stay in your own square!* Also, the different technique of body movement is reflected mainly in the procedure of shifting the weight as the steps are taken. Anyone can learn how to do this.

THE RUMBA WEIGHT SHIFT

1. With feet six inches apart, relax weight onto and over RF, Rt knee straight. Lt knee is flexed, no weight on LF.
2. Press LF to floor, straighten Lt knee as weight is pushed up into hip. Weight is now relaxed on and over LF, with RF free of weight, Rt knee flexed.
3. Press RF to floor, straighten Rt knee as weight is pushed up into hip. Weight is now relaxed on and over RF, with LF free of weight, Lt knee flexed.
4. Repeat.

An easy way to practice the Rumba weight shift is to apply the exercise when climbing a flight of stairs. If a staircase is not handy at the moment, try to emulate the pressures involved in the transfer of weight with a series of short progressive steps. Then apply the shift to the swd-close. With elevation maintained, the gradual change of weight will result in a slight sideward pelvic action. Care must be taken, though, that this reaction does not result in an exaggerated "east and west" waggle of the hips. While some hip action is intended, it should not become too obvious.

THE BASIC SOUND AND STEP PATTERN

The Rumba basic step pattern is often referred to as the *Box* or *Square*. It is not unlike the Waltz and Fox-Trot boxes, and consists of two groups of three steps each, taken within the framework of eight beats (two measures) of Rumba music in 4/4 time. The recurring sound is QQS QQS. The slow forward or backward steps are taken on the third and fourth beats of the measure—*never* on the first or second beats.

		2 measures							
	MUSIC CT.	1	2	3	4	1	2	3	4
THE	DANCE CT.	1	&	2		3	&	4	
RUMBA	DIRECTION	Swd-cl-fwd				Swd-cl-bwd			
BOX	FEET	L	R	L		R	L	R	
	SOUND	Q	Q	S		Q	Q	S	

Here again we have the familiar *three steps in quick succession* followed by a distinct pause. The directions are:

Man		Lady
Swd-cl-fwd-L-R-L	QQS	Swd-cl-bwd-R-L-R
Swd-cl-bwd-R-L-R	QQS	Swd-cl-fwd-L-R-L

When practicing with partner use the ClPos.

VARIATIONS OF THE BASIC UNIT

While the sound pattern is repetitious, the unit of movement can be altered to provide diversion from the swd-cl-fwd (or bwd), provided the result is always *three steps in quick succession!* Among the numerous step patterns made possible by changing the foot position in the unit are:

1. THE WALK. A series of three steps in quick succession, forward or backward, curving sharply to the right or left to circle around partner, or to circle out of a Break into the Arch to resume ClPos.

2. THE BREAK. Partners step away from each other on the backward steps, retaining hand clasp (man's left, lady's right). Man releases Rt hand from lady's waist. Any of the other units can be used to follow the Break.

FIRST COMBINATION

With Left Turn

COUNT	Man's Part	Lady's Part	TIME
1-&	Swd-close L-R	Swd-close R-L	Q-Q
2	Fwd L	Bwd R	S
3-&	Swd-close R-L	Swd-close L-R	Q-Q
4	Fwd R	Bwd L	S
5-&	Swd-close L-R	Swd-close R-L	Q-Q
6	Fwd L, turn Lt	Bwd R, turn Lt	S
7-&	Swd-close R-L	Swd-close L-R	Q-Q
8	Bwd R, turn Lt	Fwd L, turn Lt	S

1-&	Swd-close L-R	Swd-close R-L	Q-Q
2	Fwd L, turn Lt	Bwd R, turn Lt	S
3-&	Swd-close R-L	Swd-close L-R	Q-Q
4	Bwd R, turn Lt	Fwd L, turn Lt	S
5-&	Swd-close L-R	Swd-close R-L	Q-Q
6	Fwd L, turn Lt	Bwd R, turn Lt	S
7-&	Swd-close R-L	Swd-close L-R	Q-Q
8	Bwd R, turn Lt	Fwd L, turn Lt	S

The first 8 counts can be repeated as desired, with progress being made to LOD, by ignoring the directions to turn left on 6th and 8th counts. A complete left turn is intended on the second group of 8 counts.

Extreme care should be exercised when making the turn, to keep the feet close together, with a very short sideward movement to commence the sideward-close.

SECOND COMBINATION

Count	Man's Part	Lady's Part	Time
1-&	Swd-close L-R	Swd-close R-L	Q-Q
2	Fwd L	Bwd R	S
3-&	Swd-close R-L	Swd-close L-R	Q-Q
4	Fwd R	Bwd L	S
5-&	Swd-close L-R	Swd-close R-L	Q-Q
6	Bwd L, turn Rt	Fwd R, turn Rt	S
7-&	Swd-close R-L	Swd-close L-R	Q-Q
8	Fwd R, turn Rt	Bwd L, turn Rt	S
1-&	Swd-close L-R	Swd-close R-L	Q-Q
2	Bwd L, turn Rt	Fwd R, turn Rt	S
3-&	Swd-close R-L	Swd-close L-R	Q-Q
4	Fwd R, turn Rt	Bwd L, turn Rt	S

5-&	Swd-close L-R	Swd-close R-L	Q-Q
6	Bwd L, turn Rt	Fwd R, turn R	S
7-&	Swd-close R-L	Swd-close L-R	Q-Q
8	Fwd R, turn Rt	Bwd L, turn Rt	S

Rumba turns should be made with a gradual, rather than a sharp turning movement. When done in this manner more time is used and more steps are required than in Fox-Trot and Waltz turns; hence the turns can be commenced on the 6th count of the first group in both the 1st and 2nd combinations.

THIRD COMBINATION

COUNT	Man's Part	Lady's Part	TIME
1-&	Swd-close L-R	Swd-close R-L	Q-Q
2	Fwd L	Bwd R	S
3-&	Swd-close R-L	Swd-close L-R	Q-Q
4	Fwd R	Bwd L	S
5-&	Swd-close L-R	Swd-close R-L	Q-Q
6	Bwd L	Bwd R	S
7-&	Swd-close R-L	Swd-close L-R	Q-Q
8	Fwd R	Fwd L	S

Repeat as desired, or combine with:

1-&	Swd-close L-R	Swd-close R-L	Q-Q
2	Fwd L	Bwd R	S
3-&	Swd-close R-L	Swd-close L-R	Q-Q
4	Bwd R	Bwd L	S
5-&	Swd-close L-R	Swd-close R-L	Q-Q
6	Fwd L	Fwd R	S
7-&	Swd-close R-L	Swd-close L-R	Q-Q
8	Fwd R	Bwd L	S

Note that on the 6th count of first group both partners step *backward*, drawing away from each other. The man's left and his partner's right hand remain clasped, while his right and her left hand become disengaged but with *arms held up*. On 8th count partners resume original position.

On the 4th count of the second group partners again draw away from each other with a backward step, resuming original position on 8th count.

FOURTH COMBINATION

COUNT	Man's Part	Lady's Part	TIME
1-&	Swd-close L-R	Swd-close R-L	Q-Q
2	Fwd L	Bwd R	S
3-&	Swd-close R-L	Swd-close L-R	Q-Q
4	Bwd R	Fwd L	S
5-&	Swd-close L-R	Swd-close R-L	Q-Q
6	Bwd L	Bwd R	S
7-&	Swd-close R-L	Swd-close L-R	Q-Q
8	SIP on R	Fwd L	S
1-&	SIP on L-R	Fwd R-L	Q-Q
2	SIP on L	Fwd R	S
3-&	SIP on R-L	Fwd L-R	Q-Q
4	SIP on R	Fwd L	S
5-&	SIP on L-R	Fwd R-L	Q-Q
6	SIP on L	Fwd R	S
7-&	Swd-close R-L	Swd-close L-R	Q-Q
8	Fwd R	Bwd L	S

Again the partners move away from each other on the 6th count, this time in preparation for the lady to circle the man, thus: from the 8th count of the first group through the 6th count of the second group the man's steps are taken "in place," while the lady performs a complete circle, moving *forward* to his right side and around the man to end in original position on the 7th count. As the man commences his *in place* movements he shifts her right hand to his right hand, and as she circles around him he reaches behind him and again takes her right in his left hand to guide her to original position.

The Tango

The Tango was originally a Gypsy dance. It came to America via the Argentine Republic in the early 1900's, the era that saw ballroom dancing at its lowest ebb. These were the days of Ragtime rhythms, with dances such as the Bunny Hug and Turkey Trot dominating the scene. The One-Step and the Two-Step were at their zeniths, but, as interpreted by many, did little to improve the situation.

Along came the Argentine Tango—and Vernon and Irene Castle. To this couple, America's first ballroom dance team, must be given the credit for stemming the tide of extreme vulgarity in ballroom, or dance-hall, dancing. Their career together was short, as Vernon Castle was one of the first American airmen to lose his life in World War I.

The Tango today is different from that of 1914, but it has retained the same basic elements. The music is written in 2/4 and 4/4 time, and the sound is developed with slow and quick steps, as in the Fox-Trot and Rumba; but the relationship between the dances ends right there! The Tango has its own individual sound effect, or pattern, because of the timing sequence of the closing and draw steps. A common error is the application of Fox-Trot timing to this element, which tends to destroy any semblance of the Tango.

One of the Tango's chief characteristics is the sound effect of the Tango-Close unit. The familiar *three steps in quick succession,* followed by a distinct pause is again present, but this time the pause is made with the foot in the DRAW position, instead of forward or backward as in the Fox-Trot and Rumba.

Sound and Step Pattern for Closed and Promenade Basic

To dance with a partner, start in ClPos. On the first Tango-Close the man prepares to lead into PromPos; on the second he leads into ClPos.

(Closed Basic—2 Measures)

MUSIC CT.	1	2	3	4	1	2	3	4
DANCE CT.	1		2		3	&	4	
Man	L		R		L —	R —	L	
	fwd		fwd		fwd-swd-draw			
DIRECTION								
	bwd		bwd		bwd-swd-draw			
Lady	R		L		R —	L —	R	
SOUND	S		S		Q —	Q —	S	

(PromPos Basic—2 Measures)

MUSIC CT.	1	2	3	4	1	2	3	4
DANCE CT.	1		2		3	&	4	
Man	L		R		L —	R —	L	
	Swd		cross		fwd-swd-draw			
DIRECTION								
	Swd		cross		bwd-swd-draw			
Lady	R		L		R —	L —	R	
SOUND	S		S		Q —	Q —	S	

Man's Lt and lady's Rt shoulder contact should be maintained in PromPos; lady turns head slightly to look toward LOD while in PromPos, then resumes full ClPos.

SOUND AND STEP VARIATION

In addition to the Tango-Close there are the Habanera, the Rock, and the Tango Cross. Each has identical timing: QQS. Except for the Tango-Close, the other units consist of but three changes of weight. The Habanera is basically a rocking movement: bwd or fwd. Progress to LOD is made with a series in either direction. When alternated, spot turns can be made to Rt or Lt. Habaneras can be started on either foot to either direction, man or lady alternating, hence the foot used to start is not indicated.

Habanera Forward

Rock fwd, SIP bwd, SIP fwd QQS

Habanera Backward

Rock bwd, SIP fwd, SIP bwd

Figure 24

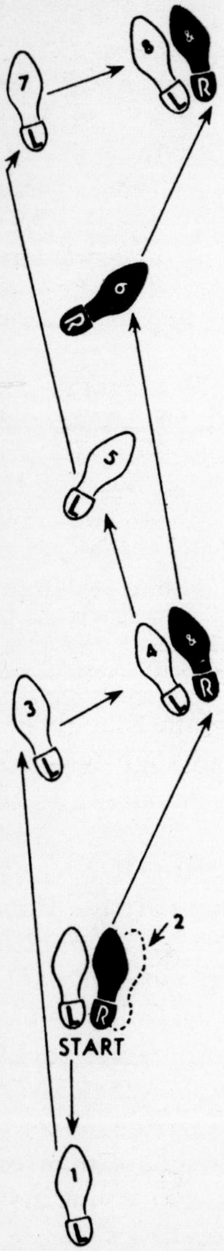

FIRST COMBINATION

Man's Part

COUNT		TIME
1	Cortez bwd L....	S
2	Fwd R, ...	S
3-&	Fwd L—swd R..	Q-Q
4	Draw L to R, no weight on L....	S
	Repeat from 1st count as desired, or combine with:	
5	Swd (or diagonally fwd) L....	S
6	Cross R between self and partner	S
7-&	Fwd L—swd R...	Q-Q
8	Draw L to R, no weight on L...	S

Repeat from 5th count as desired, or combine with first 4 counts.

Figure 25

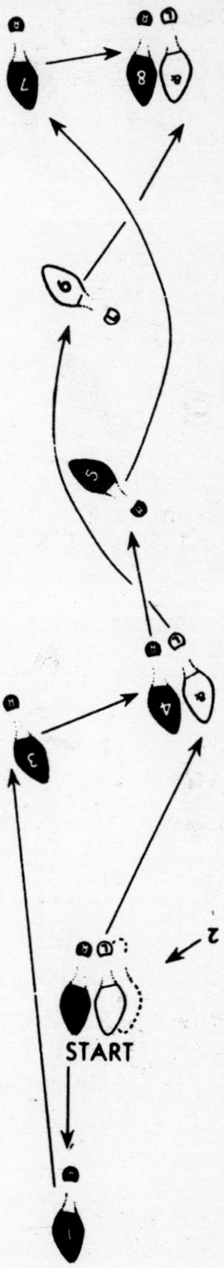

FIRST COMBINATION

Lady's Part

COUNT		TIME
1	Cortez fwd R....	S
2	Bwd L.........	S
3-&	Bwd R—swd L..	Q-Q
4	Draw R to L, no weight on R...	S
	Repeat from 1st count as desired, or combine with:	
5	Swd (or diagonally bwd) R...	S
6	Cross L between self and partner	S
7-&	Bwd R—swd L..	Q-Q
8	Draw R to L, no weight on R...	S

Repeat from 5th count as desired, or combine with first 4 counts.

Figure 26

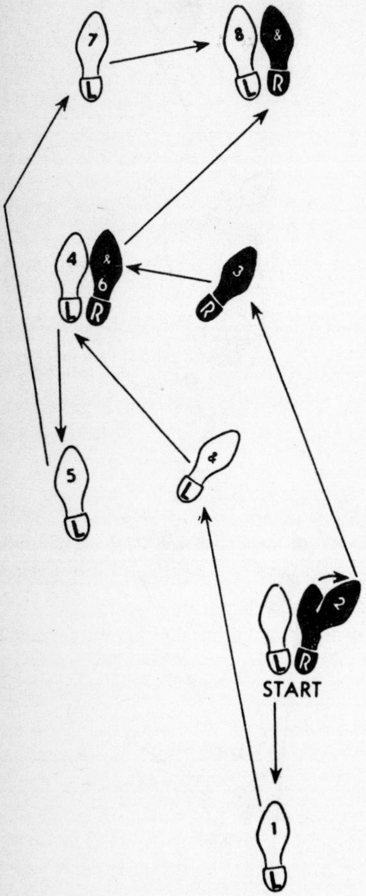

SECOND COMBINATION

Man's Part

COUNT		TIME
1	Cortez bwd L. . . .	S
2-&	Fwd R—swd L. . .	Q-Q
3	Cross R between self and partner	S
4-&	Swd-close L-R. . .	Q-Q
5	Cortez bwd L. . . .	S
6	Fwd R.	S
7-&	Fwd L—swd R. .	Q-Q
8	Draw L to R, no weight on L. . .	S

Repeat as desired from 1st count.

SECOND COMBINATION

Lady's Part

COUNT		TIME
1	Cortez fwd R....	S
2-&	Bwd L—swd R ..	Q-Q
3	Cross L between self and partner	S
4-&	Swd-close R-L...	Q-Q
5	Cortez fwd R....	S
6	Bwd L..........	S
7-&	Bwd R—swd L ..	Q-Q
8	Draw R to L, no weight on R...	S

Repeat as desired from 1st count.

Figure 27

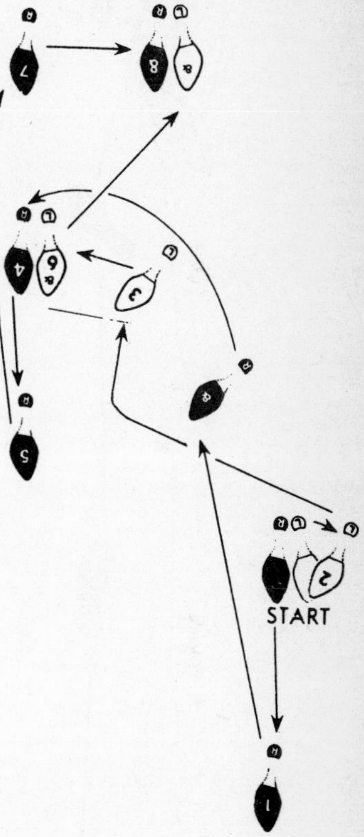

Figure 28

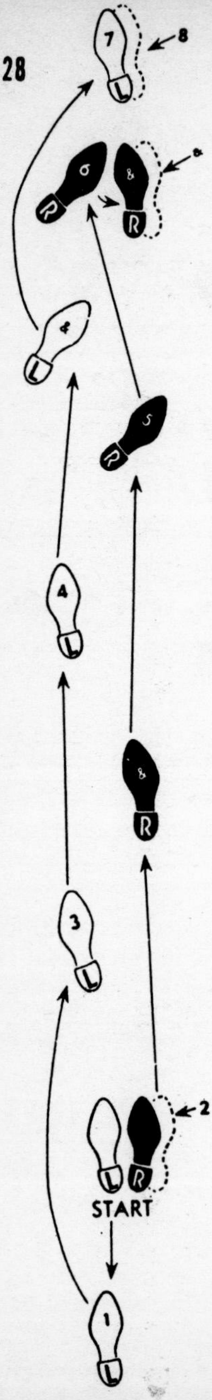

THIRD COMBINATION

Man's Part

COUNT		TIME
1	Cortez bwd L....	S
2	Fwd R.........	S
3-&	Fwd L-R.......	Q-Q
4	Fwd L..........	S
5-&	Fwd R—swd L..	Q-Q
6	Cross R between self and partner	S
7-&	Rock fwd L—bwd R...........	Q-Q
8-&	Rock fwd L—bwd R...........	Q-Q

Repeat as desired from 1st count.

Figure 29

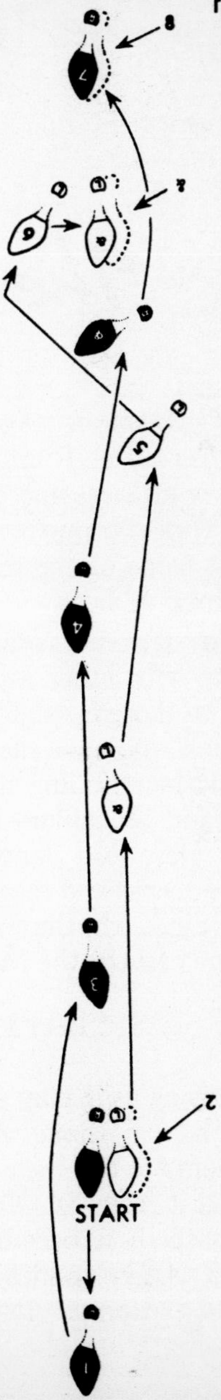

THIRD COMBINATION

Lady's Part

COUNT		TIME
1	Cortez fwd R. . . .	S
2	Bwd L.	S
3-&	Bwd R-L.	Q-Q
4	Bwd R.	S
5-&	Bwd L—swd R. .	Q-Q
6	Cross L between self and partner	S
7-&	Rock bwd R — fwd L.	Q-Q
8-&	Rock bwd R — fwd L.	Q-Q

Repeat as desired from 1st count.

The Mambo

THE MAMBO is a syncopated adaptation of the Cuban Bolero and Rumba. In its original form, Mambo is wild, free, and expressive, spiced with the jungle-like rhythm of primitive rituals and folk dance movements. At least some of the original characteristics are retained by Mambo addicts.

Removed from its original habitat, Mambo at once takes its place with other accepted social dances. This is due largely to those far-sighted members of the dance teaching profession who have succeeded in standardizing a modified form of this thrilling dance. To thousands of people—young and old alike—Mambo offers a tantalizing challenge. Here is a dance which demands a maximum of rhythmic sense and response—especially on the part of the lady. Since rhythm and response can be developed, everyone can try the Mambo.

BASIC RHYTHM AND PATTERN

Surprising as it may seem to the uninitiated, Mambo is based on a rhythmic sequence consisting of but six foot movements to two measures (8 beats) of music. It sounds easy and it really is. Once the rhythmic motion has been accomplished, it becomes comparatively easy to change the step pattern to include breaks, commandos, and other standard patterns. It is interesting to note that all the varied positions are used in Mambo: closed position (Cl-Pos), open break position (OB-Pos), challenge position (Ch-Pos) and conversational position (Con-Pos). (*See* Terms and Abbreviations, pp. 1-2.)

Remember that the feet are never brought to the closed position in what is termed the basic step; rather, they are consistently in either a *forward*, *backward*, or *sideward* open position. Also, on the movement Press R bwd, the heel must not be lowered to the floor. (*See* Terms and Abbreviations, pp. 1-2.) On this same step the knee may be slightly bent as the ball of foot receives the weight, but it must not bend after the transfer of weight.

First Half

			Dance Movement	
Measure	Time	Dance Count	**Man's Part**	**Lady's Part**
1	S	4–1	Bwd L	Fwd R
	Q	2	Press R bwd	Press L fwd
	Q	3	SIP L	SIP R

Second Half

2	S	4–1	Fwd R	Bwd L
	Q	2	Press L fwd	Press R bwd
	Q	3	SIP R	SIP L

The first step in each half is counted 4–1. This indicates the last and first beats, respectively, of two succeeding measures of music. In execution, the first step in each half is anticipated; that is, it is started on the last beat of a preceding measure and held through the first beat of the following measure. With each increase in tempo there is, among Mambo fans, a tendency to complete the anticipated step closer and closer to the first beat. This sets up a distinctive rhythm which characterizes Mambo. The same step pattern, danced within the framework of each succeeding measure (1–2, 3, 4, 1–2, 3, 4) somehow fails to meet head-on the challenge hurled by well-regulated Mambo music.

A close study of the foregoing will acquaint the student of Mambo with one of its chief characteristics: the constant repetition of the basic rhythmic sequence. Everything else the dancer does can change—step pattern, body position, etc.—but the rhythmic sequence must never vary from what a beginner in Mambo might be tempted to refer to as "monotonous repetition."

Man's Part	TIME	DANCE COUNT	Lady's Part
L	S	4–1	R
R	Q	2	L
L	Q	3	R
R	S	4–1	L
L	Q	2	R
R	Q	3	L

Diligent practice may be required before the movement becomes automatic and variations follow one another in perfect timing. A common fault is to execute two slow steps in succession at any given point in the pattern. This destroys the basic rhythm and should be corrected immediately.

As early as possible, an attempt should be made to make a left turn while doing the basic step. The man can do this by keeping his glance toward the left and by bearing in that direction.

Although the Mambo is a constant repetition of the basic *slow-quick-quick* rhythmic pattern, the dancer is urged to take liberties with the step pattern, always keeping in mind that strict adherence to the framework of the rhythm is essential to a correct interpretation.

VARIATIONS IN STEP PATTERN

To change the step pattern merely change the direction of a lead step (4–1); for example, on completion of the "preparation" (first half of the basic step), step *sideward* on 4–1. This develops the pattern which is referred to as the "Cuban (or Open) Break."

The Cuban (or Open) Break

TIME	DANCE COUNT	**Man's Part**	**Lady's Part**	POSITION
		Preparation		
S	4–1	Bwd L	Fwd R	Cl-Pos
Q	2	Press R bwd	Press L fwd	Cl-Pos
Q	3	SIP	SIP R	Cl-Pos
		Break		
S	4–1	Swd R	Swd L	OB-Pos
Q	2	Press L bwd	Press R bwd	OB-Pos
Q	3	SIP R	SIP L	OB-Pos

At the beginning of the break, the man releases his hold on the lady with his right hand, so that both may step *backward* and away from each other on 2.

Turnabout and Break

The Turnabout is a movement, consisting of three steps each for the man and the lady, in which a complete but extremely tight circle is made. He circles to his left on L–R–L, and simultaneously she circles to her right on R–L–R. They face each other at the start and at the finish, and the circle described by the movement should be narrow enough in diameter to enable them to remain in close proximity. The challenge position (Ch-Pos) is used for this movement, with open break position (OB-Pos) being used on the break.

Turnabout

Man's Part		Time	Dance Count	Lady's Part	
L	Make tight	S	4–1	R	Make tight
R	circle to	Q	2	L	circle to
L	left	Q	3	R	right

Break

Man's Part	Time	Dance Count	Lady's Part
Swd R	S	4–1	Swd L
Press L bwd	Q	2	Press R bwd
SIP R	Q	3	SIP L

A sharp turn on his L on 4–1, and a pedaling movement on the ball of R to lend impetus to the turn on 2 will help the man to complete the circle within a tight radius. The lady turns sharply to her right on 4–1 and follows with a pedal-like movement on the ball of her L on 2.

It is possible to vary the above by using the challenge position throughout the entire movement.

The Commandos

In the foregoing the *closing* step (feet together) has not been used. A somewhat different expression of movement can be realized by *closing* the feet on the lead step (4–1), rather than stepping *fwd*, *bwd*, or *swd* on this beat.

Any one of the three positions, Cl-Pos, OB-Pos, Ch-Pos, can be used when doing the Commandos. Assume that a basic step has been completed, then:

Man's Part	Time	Dance Count	Lady's Part
Right Side Commando			**Left Side Commando**
Close L	S	4–1	Close R
Press R swd	Q	2	Press L swd
SIP L	Q	3	SIP R
Left Side Commando			**Right Side Commando**
Close R	S	4–1	Close L
Press L swd	Q	2	Press R swd
SIP R	Q	3	SIP L
Right Back Commando			**Left Fwd Commando**
Close L	S	4–1	Close R
Press R bwd	Q	2	Press L fwd
SIP L	Q	3	SIP R
Left Fwd Commando			**Right Back Commando**
Close R	S	4–1	Close L
Press L fwd	Q	2	Press R bwd
SIP R	Q	3	SIP L

Right Fwd Commando: on count 2 Press R fwd.
Left Bwd Commando: on count 2 Press L bwd.

TRIPLE MAMBO

The term "triple" indicates an increase in the number of steps to be taken within the framework of the measure. Instead of six steps, a total of ten steps is possible in the basic two measure Mambo phrase.

Basic Movement

Rather than actual steps, the triple movement is basically a rhythmic reaction; hence a person with slow rhythmic response will not find it easy at first.

The symbol "&" (expressed *and*) is used to count the impulse which occurs between the indicated beats of music (4 & 1). This, in turn, sets up the triple movement resulting in not one, but three steps in exactly the same musical space of time ordinarily devoted to one step.

Man's Part	Time	Dance Count	Lady's Part
Triple Bwd			**Triple Fwd**
L bwd	Slow	4	R fwd
R SIP		&	L SIP
L SIP		1	R SIP
R Press bwd	Q	2	L Press fwd
L SIP	Q	3	R SIP
Triple Fwd			**Triple Bwd**
R fwd	Slow	4	L bwd
L SIP		&	R SIP
R SIP		1	L SIP
L Press fwd	Q	2	R Press bwd
R SIP	Q	3	L SIP

Employing the Triple

Once the technique of the triple has been perfected, it can be superimposed on all Mambo step patterns. The lead step (4–1) is now more than just a *forward* and *backward* movement; it has become an instant of impulsive reaction.

The triple movement is basic, and it can be injected wherever the count 4–1 occurs, by changing the count to 4 & 1. Keep in mind that the additional movement should be thought of in terms of an *impulsive reaction* rather than steps. Also remember that injecting the triple in no way changes the musical phrasing; its length remains exactly the same.

Applied to the Commandos, this is the triple effect:

Man's Part	Time	Dance Count	Lady's Part
L close—R-L SIP	S	4 & 1	R close—L-R SIP
R Press swd (bwd)	Q	2	L Press swd (fwd)
L SIP	Q	3	R SIP
R close—L-R SIP	S	4 & 1	L close—R-L SIP
L Press swd (fwd)	Q	2	R Press swd (bwd)
R SIP	Q	3	L SIP

As indicated, the Commandos can be varied by changing the direction on count 2.

COMBINING THE STEP PATTERNS

The ability to progress from one step pattern to another increases the enjoyment to be derived from Mambo or any other dance. The suggested sequence of the step patterns described here is just one of the dozens used to interpret this new and fascinating rhythm.

Man's Part	Dance Count	Lady's Part
1. Basic Step	4–1, 2, 3, 4–1, 2, 3	Same
2. Cuban Break	4–1, 2, 3, 4–1, 2, 3	Same
3. Turnabout & Break	4–1, 2, 3, 4–1, 2, 3	Same
4. Rt. fwd Commando	4–1, 2, 3	Lt. bwd Commando
Lt. bwd Commando	4–1, 2, 3	Rt. fwd Commando
5. Rt. swd Commando	4–1, 2, 3	Lt. swd Commando
Lt. swd Commando	4–1, 2, 3	Rt. swd Commando
6. Rt. fwd Commando	4–1, 2, 3	Turnabout
Break	4–1, 2, 3	Same

The Samba

THE Samba is quite the liveliest of the ballroom dances introduced to the United States from Latin America. Its music possesses a rollicking rhythm which suggests a style of movement that can become as boisterous as any created by north-of-the-border jive!

The basic step pattern consists of the same movements learned in the Fox-Trot and Waltz: *fwd-swd-close . . . bwd-swd-close*. The timing is different from either of these dances and must be closely adhered to in sequence: *quick-quick-slow . . . quick-quick-slow*.

THE BASIC STEP PATTERN AND TIMING EFFECT

Measure	Music Count	Dance Movement: Left Turn	Dance Movement: Right Turn	Dance Count	Time
1	1	Fwd L	Fwd R	1	Q
	2	Swd R	Swd L	&	Q
	3–4	Close L	Close R	2	S
2	1	Bwd R	Bwd L	3	Q
	2	Swd L	Swd R	&	Q
	3–4	Close R	Close L	4	S

Note particularly that it is on the *closing* step that the pause is effected—not on the forward and backward steps as in the Fox-Trot and Rumba. This is one of the distinguishing features of the Samba and must be strictly adhered to, else the result will resemble a mixture of the Fox-Trot and Rumba.

In performing the basic steps described above, partners may assume the position used in the Rumba. The rhythmical reaction which provides Samba style can best be explained as: DOWN-up-DOWN . .. DOWN-up-DOWN. On the forward step the movement of the body is accented *downward;* on the sideward step, *upward;* on the closing step, *downward.*

The sideward step is taken on the ball of the foot, and with the quick closing step a ball-change is effected, resulting in a movement described as: *step-ball-change . . . step-ball-change.* At times the "change" is not a closing step at all; rather, it becomes an accented movement of the foot "in place."

FIRST COMBINATION

COUNT	Man's Part	Lady's Part	TIME
1	Fwd L	Bwd R	Q
&-2	Swd-close R-L	Swd-close L-R	Q-S
3	Bwd R	Bwd L	Q
&-4	Swd-close L-R	Swd-close R-L	Q-S
5	Fwd L	Bwd R	Q
&-6	Swd-close R-L	Swd-close L-R	Q-Q
&-7	Swd-close R-L	Swd-close L-R	Q-Q
&-8	Swd-close R-L	Swd-close L-R	Q-S
1	Fwd R	Bwd L	Q
&-2	Swd-close L-R	Swd-close R-L	Q-S
3	Bwd L	Fwd R	Q
&-4	Swd-close R-L	Swd-close L-R	Q-S
5	Fwd R	Bwd L	Q
&-6	Swd-close L-R	Swd-close R-L	Q-Q
&-7	Swd-close L-R	Swd-close R-L	Q-Q
&-8	Swd-close L-R	Swd-close R-L	Q-S

Repeat as desired from 1st count.

Partners may assume the closed or the Rumba position when dancing the above combination.

SECOND COMBINATION

In this combination the ball-change is used to effect the

"paddle-turn," with the sideward step serving as the paddle which helps to make complete left or right turns in four counts.

At the beginning the man lets go his hold on the lady, and each performs the paddle-turn individually, the man turning to his *left* as the lady turns to her *right*, and vice versa.

COUNT	Man's Part	Lady's Part	TIME
1	Fwd L, turn sharply *left* to face center	Fwd R, turn sharply *right* to face center	Q
&	Press ball of R swd	Press ball of L swd	Q
2	SIP on L, pivoting to face opposite LOD	SIP on R, pivoting to face LOD	Q
&	Press ball of R swd	Press ball of L swd	Q
3	SIP on L, pivoting to face wall	SIP on R, pivoting to face wall	Q
&	Press ball of R swd	Press ball of L swd	Q
4	SIP on L, pivoting to face LOD and partner	SIP on R, pivoting to face opposite LOD and partner	S
5	Fwd R, turn sharply *right* to face wall	Fwd L, turn sharply *left* to face wall	Q
&	Press ball of L swd	Press ball of R swd	Q
6	SIP on R, pivoting to face opposite LOD, back to partner	SIP on L, pivoting to face LOD, back to partner	Q
&	Press ball of L swd	Press ball of R swd	Q
7	SIP on R, pivoting to face center	SIP on L, pivoting to face center	Q
&	Press ball of L swd	Press ball of R swd	Q
8	SIP on R, pivoting to face LOD and partner	SIP on L, pivoting to face opposite LOD and partner	S

Repeat or combine with 1st combination.

Note that partners are back to back on 2nd and 6th counts.

The Merengue

The Merengue (say Me-reeng-ay) is a product of the Caribbean. It received a most enthusiastic welcome in the United States in the mid 1950's. Whether it originated in Haiti or the Dominican Republic is debatable; both countries claim credit for its inception. One legend has it that a high-ranking military figure of the Dominican Republic, his right leg stiffened from battle wounds, was the guest of honor at an official ball. Accepting the honor of leading off in the first dance, the best he could do was a repeated sideward-close in a lame-duck fashion because of his injured leg. The other guests courteously emulated his movement, thus creating a new dance. According to the Haitian legend, the crippled son of an early ruler was compelled to drag his lame leg when dancing, thus creating the style among his followers that resulted in the Merengue. Whichever legend is correct, the fact remains that the dance still retains a bit of a drag on the closing step.

Stripped of the exaggerated body sway from side-to-side that marked its early appearance, the Merengue became one of the suavest and most sophisticated dances since the Tango. As in other dances of Caribbean origin, the manner in which the weight is shifted from one foot to another marks its underlying style and technique. A slight but noticeble drag of the feet on the closing step is characteristic of the dance and dominates its technique.

The music is written in 2/4 time. The steps are made successively on each beat of music; eight steps equal eight counts or four measures. Slow and quick steps are not involved.

THE MERENGUE PROMENADE

The Merengue Promenade is a series of swd-close steps, with the dancers progressing toward LOD. In Cl-Pos, the man faces the wall, and the lady faces center.

Man:	L	R	L	R	L	R	L	R
	Swd-close		Swd-close		Swd-close		Swd-close	
Lady:	R	L	R	L	R	L	R	L
COUNT:	&1	&2	&3	&4	&5	&6	&7	&8

THE OPEN BREAK

Man:	Fwd L-R-L-R-L	&1&2&3&4&5
	Bwd (in place) R, swd-close L-R	&6&7&8
Lady:	Bwd R-L-R-L-R	&1&2&3&4&5
	Bwd L, swd-close R-L	&6&7&8

Start in Cl-Pos; on count "&6," both step bwd to OB-Pos. Do traveling steps (counts "&1"-"5") in a small circle.

THE ARCH

Man: Swd-close L-R-L-R (OB-Pos), Lt hand held high. Repeat in Cl-Pos ("&1"-"8").

Lady: Circle under man's Lt arm, do Fwd R-L-R-L. In Cl-Pos, do Swd-close R-L-R-L ("&1"-"8").

This pattern may also be started in Cl-Pos.

THE LEFT TURN

Man:	Fwd L	Bwd R	Swd-close	L	R	—Repeat
COUNT:	&1	&2		&3	&4	&5&6&7&8
Lady:	Bwd R	Fwd L	Swd-close	R	L	—Repeat

Repeat the above ("&1"-"16") to do a full turn.

THE SIDE BREAK

Man:	Fwd L, swd R, X L bwd, SIP R	&1&2&3&4
	Swd-close L-R-L-R	&5&6&7&8
Lady:	Bwd R, swd L, X R bwd, SIP L	&1&2&3&4
	Swd-close R-L-R-L	&5&6&7&8

American Swing

SINCE the 1920's, a number of bouncy, swingy dance movements have developed, all danced to a lively version of the familiar Fox-Trot rhythm. Over the years, these bouncy steps have been known variously as the Lindy, Jitterbug, Jump, Jive, Boogie, Rock 'n Roll, etc. Although strictly American in origin, these dances eventually became internationally popular, and collectively they are referred to as American Swing.

The original music and the dance to fit its temperament were first heard and seen at the old Savoy Ballroom, in New York City's Harlem. The year was 1927, when Charles Lindbergh made his famous flight over the Atlantic Ocean. To honor him, the Savoy habitués promptly named their new dance the *Lindy Hop*! If the music was a bit wild (for that era) the dance was more so. Its exaggerated style kept it in disrepute for several years, and it was only through the untiring efforts of the more progressive dance teacher organizations that it was finally modified and made acceptable to dancers of all ages, from exuberant teen-agers to mature sophisticates.

Depending upon the mood and ability of the individual, Swing can be applied to most of the livelier Fox-Trot tempos. So on your toes, everybody—and *Let's Swing It!*

SWING SOUND AND STEP PATTERN

Swing music is characterized by a heavy accent on the 2nd and 4th beats, in contrast to the softer accent on the 1st and 3rd beats of the measure in the more conventional Fox-Trot rhythm. The basic sound of Swing is *slow—slow—quick-quick.*

The basic step pattern can be described as a forward and backward step, followed by a ball-change, with a rocking motion applied. Variations of the basic step can result in three distinct sound and step patterns: the Single, Double, and Triple Swing.

The Single Sound Pattern

(1½ measures)

MUSIC	1	2	3	4	5	6	
DANCE	1	2	3	4	5	6	
Man:	L		R		L - R		
	step		step		ball-ch		*Repeat*
Lady:	R		L		R - L		
SOUND	S		S		Q - Q		

The Single Step Pattern

Man's Part	TIME	**Lady's Part**
Fwd on L	S	Fwd on R
Bwd on R (SIP)	S	Bwd on L (SIP)
Bwd on L } ball	Q	Bwd on R } ball
Fwd on R } ch	Q	Fwd on L } ch

Repeat as desired from start.

Note that only four steps are required for the Single Step unit. This unit should be practiced to develop directions and musical framework, which are identical for the Double and Triple as well.

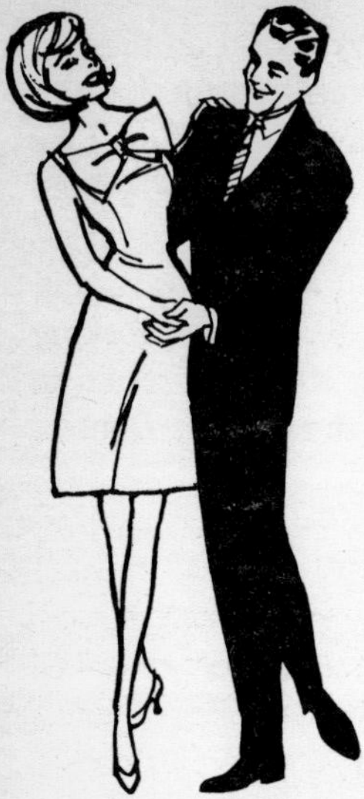

Figure 30
Basic Step in
Promenade Position

The Double Sound Pattern

In the Double sound, a tap of the foot *precedes* the shift of weight to that foot. This results in *six* sounds instead of *four,* as in the Single unit.

(1½ measures)

MUSIC	1	2	3	4	5	6	
DANCE	1	2	3	4	5	6	
Man:	L	L	R	R	L - R		
	tap	step	tap	step	ball-ch		*Repeat*
Lady:	R	R	L	L	R - L		
SOUND	SLOW		SLOW		Q - Q		

Note that the Double sound is produced in exactly the same musical framework as the Single sound.

The Double Step Pattern

Man	Dance Movement	Time		Lady
L	Tap fwd	1	S	R
L	Step fwd	2		R
R	Tap bwd	3	S	L
R	Step bwd	4		L
L	Step bwd ball	5	Q	R
R	Step fwd ch	6	Q	L

Repeat as desired from start.

TRIPLE SWING

The term "Triple" describes a sound which can be applied to Swing, Mambo, and Cha Cha. It indicates the number of movements possible within the prescribed musical framework; it also makes necessary a different method of expressing the dance count, since some of the movements must be made *between the beats* in order to increase to *eight* the number of steps, or impulses, which will now take place within the framework of six beats.

For instance, in the same time consumed for the tap-step (2 sounds) in the Double, there is set up a *step-ball-change* (3 sounds) on the same 2 beats of music. As a result, the numerical sequence of the music and dance count remains the same, but the movement which occurs *between the beats* is expressed "&" (say *and*).

Triple Sound Pattern

(1½ measures)

Music	1		2	3		4	5 6	
Dance	1	&	2	3	&	4	5-6	
Man:	L	R	L	R	L	R	L-R	
	step-ball-ch			step-ball-ch			ball-ch	*Repeat*
Lady:	R	L	R	L	R	L	R-L	
Sound	SLOW			SLOW			Q-Q	

The Triple Step Pattern

Man's Part	Dance Count		Time	Lady's Part
Fwd L	1	step	S	Fwd R
Bwd R	&	ball	L O	Bwd L
Fwd L	2	ch	W	Fwd R
Bwd R	3	step	S	Bwd L
Fwd L	&	ball	L O	Fwd R
Bwd R	4	ch	W	Bwd L
Bwd L	5	ball	Q	Bwd R
Fwd R	6	ch	Q	Fwd L

The Con-Pos or the Prom-Pos can be used to develop the Sound and Step patterns of the Triple. Relatively short steps should be used. When used in the Cl-Pos, the pattern becomes a swd-close-swd movement of the feet in the Triple.

The Breakaway and the Pushaway can be made from the Cl-Pos, with partners moving away from each other on the 2nd Triple and following with the ball-change (bwd-fwd) on 5-6.

SWING FIGURES AND VARIATIONS

Once the knack of applying the correct sound to the step patterns has been achieved, many variations applicable to Swing will be suggested. These will include:

1. *The Arch.* The lady makes a complete circle to her ***right***

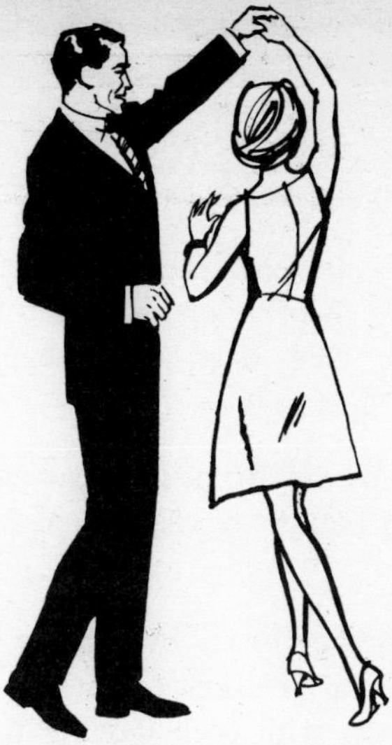

Figure 31
The Arch

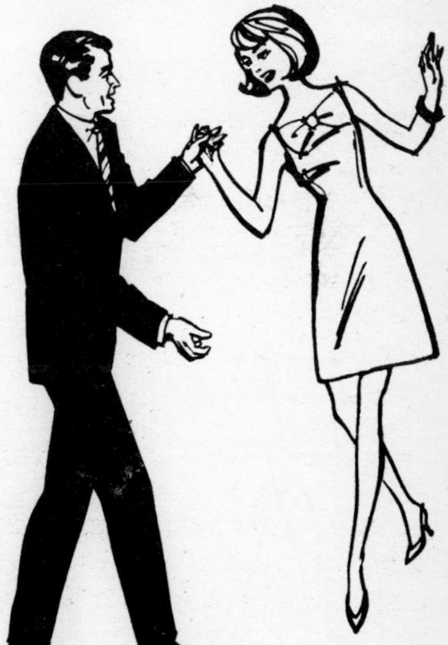

Figure 32
The Breakaway

to pass under the arch made by the raising of the man's left and her right hands.

2. *The Loop.* The lady makes a complete circle to her *left,* passing under the loop made by raising hands as in the Arch.

3. *The Breakaway.* The partners step backward away from each other. This can follow an Arch or Loop, or it can be done from Cl-Pos or Prom-Pos. Each does a ball-change (bwd-fwd) on 5-6.

4. *The Pushaway.* From Cl-Pos or Prom-Pos partners back away from each other. Both hands are clasped. Movement same as Breakaway.

5. *Change Places,* or *Double Break.* From Breakaway or Pushaway, partners take hand-shake position (right hands joined). Man leads lady into Loop with each moving into space occupied by the other at start. Both end facing each other on ball-change (5-6) and shift to normal hand-clasp.

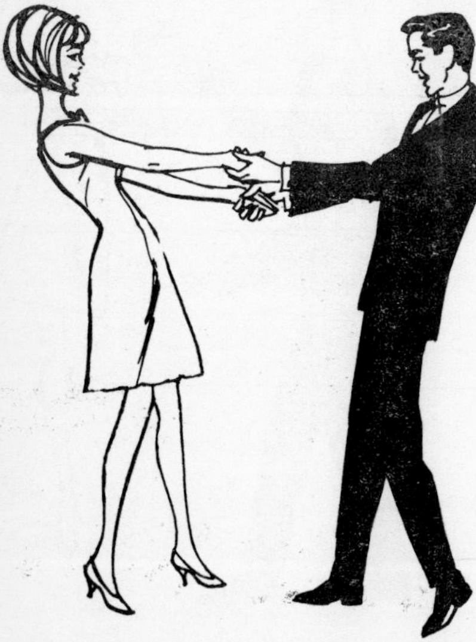

Figure 33
The Pushaway

MORE TIMELY HINTS

Perfect timing is the goal of those who aspire to extra fun and enjoyment in dancing. An occasional check of the following will help increase enjoyment of the Swing:

a. Each step pattern must be started and completed within the framework of 6 beats of music. This applies to Single, Double, and Triple.

b. A deviation by either partner from the correct timing and step sequence results in stepping on the wrong foot, with one partner being out of step with the other.

c. Except when the Sugarfoot (a twisting motion on the balls of the feet) is applied, a ball-change (bwd-fwd) is always made on counts 5-6.

d. Finally, always keep in mind this important factor regarding Swing: the Single with 4 sounds, the Double with 6 sounds, and the Triple with 8 sounds are all performed within the framework of 6 beats (1½ measures).

The Cha-Cha

THE Cha-Cha is the result of a demand by the more conservative dancers for a modification of the Mambo. In response, a few of the better Latin-American bands obliged by slowing down the tempo of their music from 50 to 30 bars per minute. The dancing public asked for more of the fascinating rhythm that resulted, and soon a wave of this new and enchanting music literally filled the air.

With the slower tempo came a subtle, swaying motion to replace the heavily accented hip and torso action of Mambo, with emphasis on foot, rather than hip, movement. Like the Mambo, Cha-Cha is danced off-beat. When the music is played in its authentic rhythm, the triple impulse occurs on the 4th beat of one measure and the 1st beat of the following measure. In some orchestrations, however, this impulse is indicated on the 3rd and 4th beats, and sometimes on the 1st and 2nd beats; it is, then, not altogether a careless attitude on the part of the dancer when the triple is done on other than the count of 4-&-1.

CHA-CHA SOUND EFFECT

Each individual unit consists of five steps, danced within the framework of 4 beats of music, with each fourth step in the numerical sequence occurring *between* the 4th beat of the first measure and the 1st beat of the second measure. The fifth step in the unit is a weight shift on the 1st beat of the second measure.

Note that the triple on the music counts of 4-&-1 results in *three steps in quick succession,* followed by a distinct pause. Note also—and this is most important—that the combined length of time consumed by the steps in the sequence count of 1-2 is exactly the same as 3-4-5.

Until the sound pattern has been fully mastered, it is suggested that the feet be raised and lowered (SIP) with no attempt to form the step pattern at this time. A total of ten steps within the framework of 8 beats comprises a Cha-Cha pattern.

	(1st measure)					(2nd measure)					
MUSIC	(1)	2	3	4	&	1	2	3	4	&	(1)
STEP SEQUENCE	(5)	1	2	3	4	5	1	2	3	4	(5)
Man:	(R)	L	R	L	R	L	R	L	R	L	(R)
Lady:	(L)	R	L	R	L	R	L	R	L	R	(L)
SOUND	(cha)	STEP	step	cha-cha-cha			STEP	step	cha-cha-(cha)		

The directions in parentheses following the second measure indicate a return to and repetition of the sound started in the first measure.

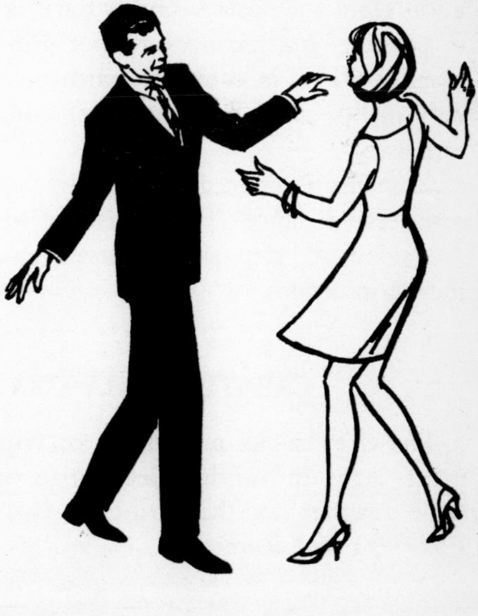

Figure 34
The Challenge Position

APPLYING SOUND TO BASIC STEP PATTERN

The first step (fwd or bwd) is made with a rocking motion. It precedes a change of direction and is emphasized slightly to check forward or backward momentum in preparation for a smooth change into the cha-cha-cha.

	(1st measure)						(2nd measure)				
MUSIC	(1)	2	3	4	&	1	2	3	4	&	(1)
STEP SEQUENCE	(5)	1	2	3	4	5	1	2	3	4	(5)
Man:	(R) (fwd)	L fwd	R bwd	L swd-	R close-	L bwd	R bwd	L fwd	R swd-	L close-	(R) (fwd)
SOUND	(cha)	STEP	step	cha-	cha-	cha	STEP	step	cha-	cha-	(cha)
Lady:	(L) (bwd)	R bwd	L fwd	R swd-	L close-	R fwd	L fwd	R bwd	L swd-	R close-	(L) (bwd)

Practice the basic step without a partner until the correct sound can be applied. When the step is danced with a partner, either Cl-Pos or Ch-Pos can be used.

Cha-Cha is a rhythm dance in the strictest sense. No deviation from the basic sound pattern is permitted. This makes it possible for partners to perform the figures in all the open positions in complete synchronization with each other's movements, since both are responding to the same rhythmic impulses.

Cha-Cha is danced in a relatively small area. It is not a progressive dance. The steps are of necessity very short; the sideward step should never be more than six to ten inches in length.

CREATING CHA-CHA FIGURES

The cha-cha-cha movement, or triple (4 & 1), is used to make turns in varying degrees to the right or left in the same manner as the swd-close-fwd or swd-close-bwd in Fox-Trot and Rumba.

The Backward Break

This is a standard pattern, also used in Rumba and Mambo; the difference is in the timing. The position is similar to the Breakaway in Swing, Figure 32, p. 69.

	Man's Part	Count	Lady's Part
a.	Fwd L, bwd R	2-3	Bwd R, fwd L
	Swd-close-bwd L-R-L	4-&-1	Swd-close-fwd R-L-R
	Bwd R, fwd L	2-3	Fwd L, bwd R
b.	Swd-close-SWD R-L-R	4-&-1	Swd-close-SWD L-R-L
c.	BWD L, fwd R	2-3	BWD R, fwd L
	Swd-close-SWD L-R-L	4-&-1	Swd-close-SWD R-L-R
d.	Bwd R, fwd L	2-3	Fwd L, bwd R
	Swd-close-fwd R-L-R	4-&-1	Swd-close-bwd L-R-L

(*a*) *In Cl-Pos.* (*b*) *Sharp SWD step, release his Rt, her Lt hand hold.* (*c*) *Step backward* away *from partner, his Lt, her Rt hands clasped.* (*d*) *Resume Cl-Pos.*

The Arch

This step is similar to the Arch in Swing, Rumba, and Mambo, with the lady making a sharp circle to her right to end facing her partner in preparation for the next pattern. See Figure 31, p. 69.

	Man's Part	Count	Lady's Part
a.	Fwd L, bwd R	2-3	Bwd R, fwd L
	Swd-close-bwd L-R-L	4-&-1	Swd-close-fwd R-L-R
	Bwd R, fwd L	2-3	Fwd L, bwd R
b.	Swd-close-SWD R-L-R	4-&-1	Swd-close-SWD L-R-L
c.	Bwd L, fwd R	2-3	Bwd R, fwd L
d.	Swd-close-SIP L-R-L	4-&-1	Fwd-fwd-fwd R-L-R
e.	Bwd R, fwd L	2-3	Bwd L, fwd R
	Swd-close-SIP R-L-R	4-&-1	Swd-close-fwd L-R-L

(*a*) *In Cl-Pos.* (*b*) *Sharp swd step, release his Rt, her Lt hand hold.* (*c*) *Step backward* away *from partner on count 2.*

(d) Man assists lady to circle under Arch to face him on 3rd fwd step. (e) Retain hand clasp and step bwd away from each other on count 2, then toward each other on count 3 to resume Cl-Pos.

The Cross Break

Start: partners face each other in Ch-Pos, but with hands joined. Man's back to center, lady's back to wall.

	Man's Part	Count	Lady's Part
a.	Fwd L, bwd R	2-3	Bwd R, fwd L
	Swd-close-bwd L-R-L	4-&-1	Swd-close-fwd R-L-R
	Bwd R, fwd L	2-3	Fwd L, bwd R
b.	Swd-close-fwd R-L-R to end facing opp LOD	4-&-1	Swd-close-fwd L-R-L to end facing opp LOD
	Fwd L, bwd R	2-3	Fwd R, bwd L
c.	Swd-close-fwd L-R-L to end facing LOD	4-&-1	Swd-close-fwd R-L-R to end facing LOD
	Fwd R, bwd L	2-3	Fwd L, bwd R
d.	Swd-close-fwd R-L-R to end facing partner	4-&-1	Swd-close-bwd L-R-L to end facing partner

(b) Man turns 1/4 Rt, lady 1/4 Lt, to face opp LOD, releasing his Rt, her Lt hands; in this side-by-side position his Lt and her Rt hands are clasped and held shoulder high.

(c) Man turns 1/2 Lt, lady 1/2 Rt to face LOD, releasing his Lt, her Rt hands; in this side-by-side position his Rt and her Lt hands are clasped and held shoulder high.

(d) Resume Cl-Pos and repeat.

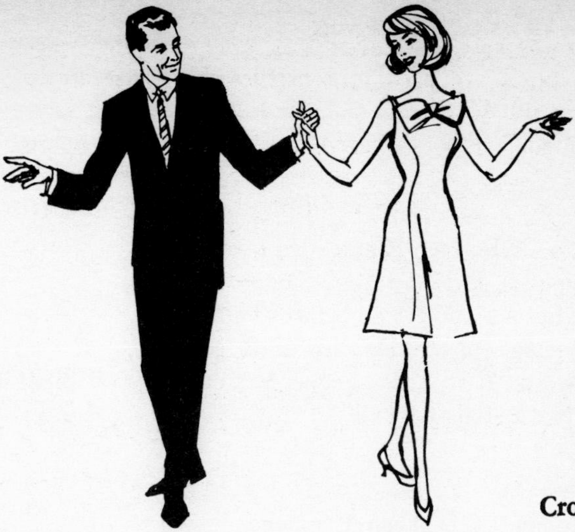

Figure 35
Cross Break (b)

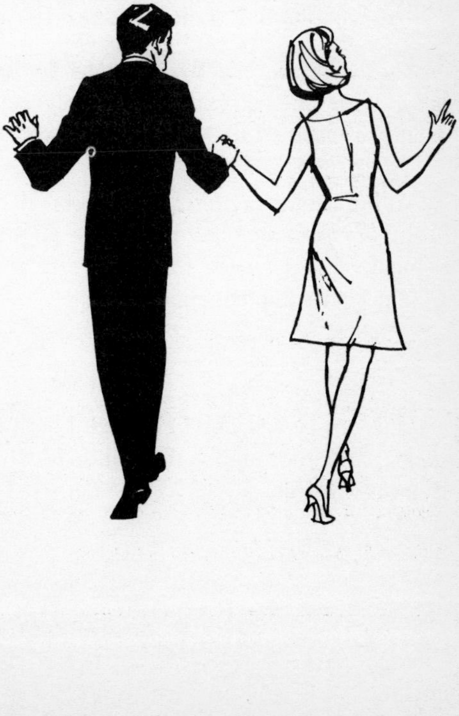

Figure 36
Cross Break (c)

The Pivots

The Pivot turns are used to construct the Chase. It is essential that a full ½ turn to right or left be made on each pivot as indicated.

The Right Pivot	COUNT
Fwd on L to LOD, keep R extended bwd with equal weight	2
Make ½ right turn (pivot) on balls of both feet to end facing opp LOD, then shift entire weight fwd on R	3
Swd-close-fwd L-R-L	4-&-1

The Left Pivot	
Fwd on R opp LOD, keep L extended bwd with equal weight	2
Make ½ left turn (pivot) on balls of both feet to end facing LOD, then shift weight fwd to L	3
Swd-close-fwd R-L-R	4-&-1

The parts are exactly the same for both the man and the lady, with one exception: the lady starts the Right Pivot facing *opposite* LOD, the Left Pivot facing *toward* LOD.

An important factor in the Pivots: the Left Pivot is started with a *forward step on the RF*; the Right Pivot is started with a *forward step on the LF*. The resultant effect of each pivot should be a complete about-face.

The Chase

This can be a tricky figure until both the man and the lady understand thoroughly their individual parts of the Pivots. Start in Ch-Pos.

	Man's Part	Count	Lady's Part
a.	Pivot Rt on L-R	2-3	Bwd R, fwd L
	Cha-cha-cha L-R-L	4-&-1	Cha-cha-cha R-L-R
b.	Pivot Lt on R-L	2-3	Pivot Rt on L-R
	Cha-cha-cha R-L-R	4-&-1	Cha-cha-cha L-R-L
c.	Fwd L, bwd R	2-3	Pivot Lt on R-L
	Cha-cha-cha L-R-L	4-&-1	Cha-cha-cha R-L-R
d.	Bwd R, fwd L	2-3	Fwd L, bwd R
	Cha-cha-cha R-L-R	4-&-1	Cha-cha-cha L-R-L

The sequence can be memorized and called as follows: (a) Man pivots. (b) Both pivot. (c) Lady pivots. (d) Neither pivots.

Discotheque Dances

Discotheque dancing can be traced back to the mid 1950's and the new sound and movements made famous by Elvis Presley. Later the Beatles and other groups began putting the accent on the second, or upbeat, of the musical measure. This brought about a radical changeover from the rhythmical intonation produced by accenting the first, or downbeat, and inspired new responses in dancing. Since so few orchestras produced the new sound and rhythm, discotheques (cabarets in which the patrons dance to recorded music) sprang up.

Disco Dances are, to many, a relief from the task of blending body movement in the contact positions required in the somewhat stereotyped patterns of the older dances. They provide the opportunity to express personal feelings by executing in solo those motions which are suggested by the music.

The basic element of Discotheque Dances is founded on the movements of the Twist; that is, *contrary body movement.* This movement is natural—in walking, the right arm and the left leg move forward together, and vice versa. (To prove how natural it is, try the bath towel routine after a shower.) It may, though, require a bit of practice to apply it successfully to musical accents. So let's Twist into Discoland!

THE TWIST

No other dance has been so appropriately titled or enjoyed as much popularity as the Twist. During its brief reign it stole the show from the previous favorites. Danced to medium-tempo, bouncy music in 4/4 time, the Twist is easy to learn. No actual steps are involved, only a minimum of inhibitions plus the wish to express oneself to rhythm.

THE BASIC TWIST

To start, stand with feet apart, LF diagonally forward. Upper arms are in natural position, forearms horizontal, palms inward. Movements are the same for both man and lady.

First Exercise	COUNT
a. Swing Rt arm bwd, Lt arm fwd..............	1
b. Swing Lt arm bwd, Rt arm fwd	2
Repeat above	3-4

Note that the Rt arm is swung backward and the Lt arm forward on the *odd,* and the Rt arm forward and the Lt arm backward on the *even* numerical counts. Head and shoulders do not turn as arms are moved.

Second Exercise	COUNT
a. On odd count, twist hips to right.............	1
b. On even count, twist hips to left..............	2
Repeat above	3-4

Note the gentle rotation of the hips as a result of this exercise. Remember: the head and shoulders do not turn. Only the hips are permitted to Twist!

On (a) Rt knee will straighten, Lt knee will flex.

On (b) Lt knee will straighten, Rt knee will flex.

Practice these exercises until the contra-movement on which the Twist is based has been developed. A slight twisting of the feet will take place thus: on the odd count (a) the heels will swivel to the right; on the even count (b) the heels will swivel to the left.

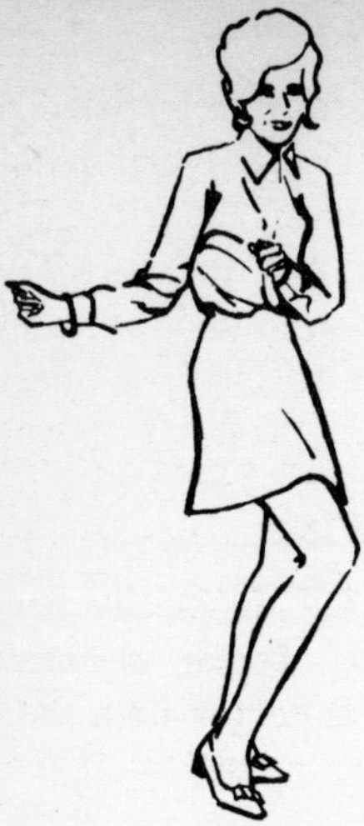

Figure 37
The Basic Twist

TWIST VARIATIONS

The Twist is basically a solo operation, hence a partner is not necessary. However, when it is danced with a partner, the man and the lady Twist on opposite feet: the man starts off on LF, the lady on RF, and they do opposite movements.

Unlike the more conventional dances, in the Twist the feet are not required to be moved in sequence to form step patterns; they remain in an open position throughout, with the hips and arms describing the Twist movements.

The Twist Rocks

	Count
a. Lean slightly fwd and Twist over LF	1-2-3-4
b. Lean slightly bwd and Twist over RF	5-6-7-8
c. Lean slightly left and Twist over LF	1-2-3-4
d. Lean slightly right and Twist over RF	5-6-7-8

The Knee Lifts

a. Lean slightly bwd on RF, flex Lt knee,
heel up, toe down, Twist on RF..............1-2-3-4
b. Lean slightly fwd on LF, flex Rt knee,
heel up, toe down, Twist on LF..............5-6-7-8

Other variations will suggest themselves as the dancer becomes more proficient in executing the basic Twist movement. A point to remember: the shoulders *do not* turn as the arms are thrust forward and backward; the twisting is from the waist downward!

Another point to remember: should soreness or stiff muscles result from practice it is a sure sign that these muscles needed the exercise . . . so just keep on twisting!

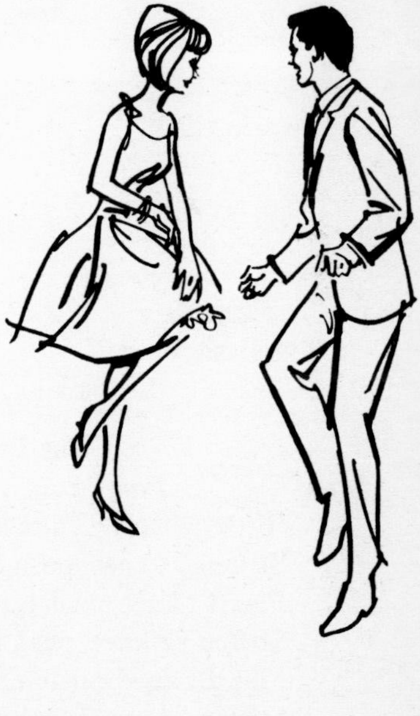

Figure 38
The Knee Lifts

THE FRUG

The Frug consists of a basic hip movement with contra-motions of the hands and arms, the latter aimed at adding zest and variety as the dance progresses. When dancing in couples, partners may face each other or stand side by side. A sequence of patterns is not necessary; however, one partner may signal the other for certain motions. There are no prescribed dance steps other than a shift of weight from one foot to the other. Since the feet play a secondary part in the Frug, it is the expression of the body to the music that is significant.

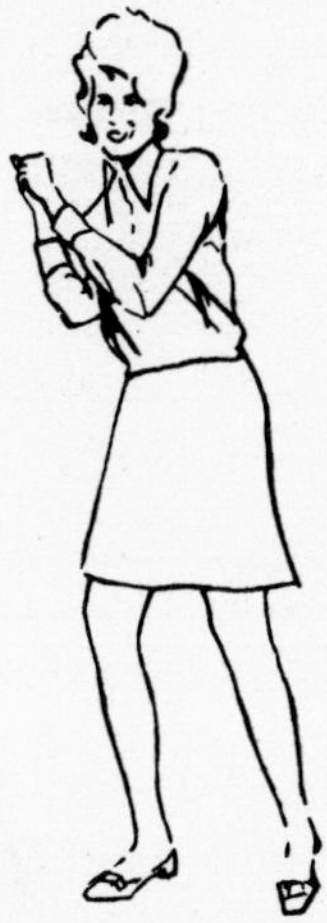

Figure 39
The Basic Frug

The Basic Frug

Meas	*Part A*	Count
1	*With wt on RF:* flex Lt knee, push hips to Rt	1
	Stiffen Lt knee, push hips to Lt	&
	Flex Lt knee, push hips to Rt	2
	Stiffen Lt knee, push hips to Lt	&
	Flex Lt knee, push hips to Rt	3
	Stiffen Lt knee, push hips to Lt	&
	Flex Lt knee, push hips to Rt	4

2	*With wt on LF:* flex Rt knee, push hips to Lt	5
	Stiffen Rt knee, push hips to Rt	&
	Flex Rt knee, push hips to Lt	6
	Stiffen Rt knee, push hips to Rt	&
	Flex Rt knee, push hips to Lt	7
	Stiffen Rt knee, push hips to Rt	&
	Flex Rt knee, push hips to Lt	8

On 1st ct. push Rt arm bwd, raise Lt arm across in front of body. On 5th ct. push Lt arm bwd, raise Rt arm across front. Note that weight is shifted to LF on ct. 5, and to RF on ct. 8.

Variations

The contramotion of the hands and arms, as developed in the basic Frug, will help to create such variations as the Stretch, the Washerwoman, the Hitchhiker, the Swim (including the various strokes), and numerous fun-producing antics!

The Washerwoman

On cts. 1-4 do the washboard motion toward the left; on cts. 5-8, toward the right.

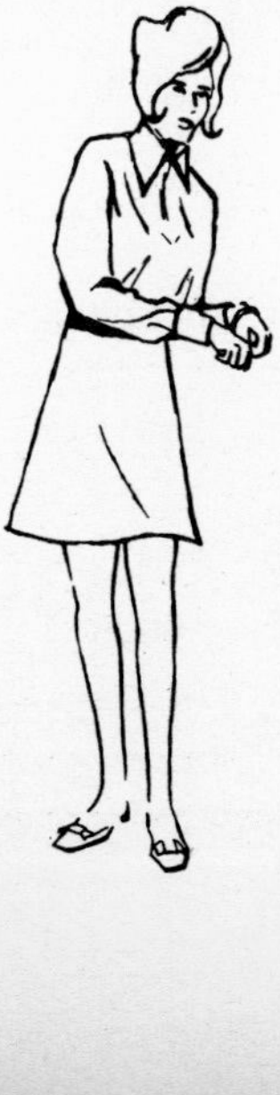

Figure 40
The Washerwoman

The Hitchhiker

On cts. 1-4, with weight on RF, use Lt arm to flag down the car. On cts. 5-8, with weight on LF, use Rt arm.

The Stretch

On cts. 1-4 stretch upward with Lt arm. On cts. 5-8 stretch upward with Rt arm.

THE WATUSI

Back in the early 1930's the Conga was one of the first Caribbean imports to become popular in the United States. Its pattern was a simple *side-cross-side-kick,* danced either in couple formation or as a single file dance with one's hands on the shoulders or hips of the person in front.

In the Watusi the same pattern is used, but with definite changes of timing and foot positions, plus hand, arm, and hip motions in compliance with the musical sound effects. It can be danced by individual couples, or with a line of boys facing a line of girls, all executing a prearranged sequence of movements.

First Variation

Meas	Boy's Part—Girl does opposite	Count
1	Swd on LF, turn body slightly to Rt	1-2
	Close RF against LF with quick motion ..	&
	Swd on LF, lean slightly to Lt	3
	Kick RF to Rt and clap hands	4
2	Swd on RF, turn slightly to Lt	5-6
	Close LF against RF with quick motion..	&
	Swd on RF, lean slightly to Rt	7
	Kick LF to Lt and clap hands	8

Second Variation

Meas	Boy's Part—Girl does opposite	Count
3	Swd on LF, turn slightly to Rt	1-2
	Cross RF behind LF with quick motion..	&
	Swd on LF	3
	Kick RF fwd to Rt and clap hands	4
4	Start with RF, reverse meas 3	5-6 & 7-8

Third Variation

5	Swd on LF, keep facing fwd	1-2
	Close RF against LF with quick motion	&
	Swd on LF	3
	Kick RF across in front of LF and clap hands	4
6	Start with RF, reverse meas 5	5-6 & 7-8

Fourth Variation

7	Swd on LF, swing both hands bwd	1-2
	Close RF against LF, swing hands upward	&
	Step in place on LF	3
	Bend Rt knee against Lt knee, clap hands	4
8	Start with RF, reverse meas 7	5-6 & 7-8

Other variations, including left and right turns, are possible with the above step patterns; however, it is suggested that every effort be made to maintain the exact sound effect.

THE BOOGALOO

This is a simple movement which can be done as a *step-tap,* a *step-brush,* or as a *step-ball-change* with the accent on counts two and four. In couple formation, partners use opposite feet.

MEAS	The Step-Tap	COUNT
1	Swd on LF, push hips to Lt	1
	Tap ball of RF against LF	2
	Swd on RF, push hips to Rt	3
	Tap ball of LF against RF	4
2	Repeat meas 1	5-8
3-4	Repeat meas 1 and 2	1-8

The Brush

1	Swd on LF, push hips to Lt	1
	Brush RF across in front of LF	2
	Swd on RF, push hips to Rt	3
	Brush LF across in front of RF	4
2	Repeat meas 1	5-8
3-4	Repeat meas 1 and 2	1-8

The Step-Ball-Change

1	Swd on Lf	1
	Press ball of RF at side of LF	&-2
	Step in place on LF	3
	Press ball of LF at side of RF	&-4
2	Repeat meas 1	5-8
	Repeat meas 1 and 2	1-8

NOTE: In each of these three step patterns, apply the following movements:

1. On counts one and two (swd to Lt) of each step, hips are thrust to Lt, with Rt arm swinging to front, Lt arm to rear.
2. On counts three and four (swd to Rt) of each step, hips are thrust to Rt, with Lt arm swinging to front, Rt arm to rear. This will develop the contramotion necessary to the styling of the Boogaloo.

THE FUNKY BROADWAY

Use the same step pattern as in the Boogaloo, but add a sharp bend of the knees on counts two, four, six, and eight. Also, the motion of the hands and arms can be exaggerated.

THE MONKEY

Stand with feet just a few inches apart, with forearms in horizontal postion in front of the body. Count one to eight (as in the other figures) and snap the hips sharply backward *on each count!* Make a complete circle with one hand on the *odd* count, and with the other hand on the *even* count.

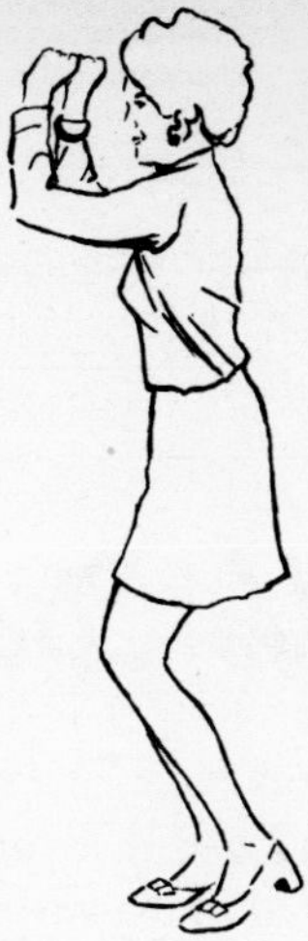

Figure 41
The Jerk

THE JERK

Start with knees flexed. Straighten knees with a snap, push hips bwd, swing arms bwd (count one). Bend knees sharply, push hips fwd, swing arms fwd (count two). Similar to The Monkey, but in slower timing.

Folk Dancing

Some Folk Dances had their origin in European countries and are closely related to the various customs and occupations of those who first danced them, many years ago. Some are of American origin, and their figures are used to create our play party dances: squares, rounds, longways, circles. To many people, Folk Dancing is something to watch, but not to do; to many others it is an outlet for personal exuberance, a means of fostering sociability and getting together groups of active people, young and old, with the aim of setting to rhythm the fundamentals of physical coordination.

As in Square Dancing, the figures are prearranged sequences of basic movements of the feet and body set to music. Many of the basic foot movements in Folk Dances are derived from the Polka, the Schottische, and the Two-Step, which are done to music in 2/4 time, and the Mazurka and Waltz, done in 3/4 time. Again as in Square Dancing, once the step patterns have been mastered the reaction to the music being played will help to create in the dancer the styles of the various numbers. As compared to regular ballroom dancing, in Folk Dancing there is very little actual body contact of the partners involved; as a consequence, there is a minimum of leading and following.

The procedures used in mastering a Folk Dance are the same as those applied in other types of dances. First of all, get the *feel* of the music by moving the feet forward or in a circle and, at times, clapping the hands in rhythmic sequence; second, learn the step pattern *without* a partner; third, take a partner and start to dance!

THE VARSOUVIENNE

Some say this dance originated in France, others claim Poland as its home, while many would like us to believe it got its start near Mt. Vesuvius in Italy. The fact is, though, that Americans of Swedish ancestry gave it quite a push several years ago, so let's give Sweden the credit. While it is one of the more sedate types of Folk Dances, the inclusion of standard Waltz steps might render it slightly more technical.

To start, form a circle of couples facing LOD. Pårtners take the PromPos: girl at boy's right, her Lt arm extended across in front of boy, Lt hands joined. His Rt arm is extended across her back, Rt hands joined. *Both start with LF!*

First Part

Meas		Count
1	Both take 3 steps (L-R-L), change positions by girl passing in front of boy. Girl is now at boy's Lt side	1-2-3
2	Both extend RF, heel down, toe up, no wt	4-5-6
3	Both take 3 steps (R-L-R), change to first postion	1-2-3
4	Both extend LF, heel down, toe up, no wt	4-5-6
5-8	Repeat the entire 1st four meas	12 cts.
9-10	Both fwd-close L-R, then hop on R and repeat	1-6
11-12	Repeat meas 1-2 to change positions	1-6
13-14	Both fwd-close R-L, then hop on L and repeat	1-6
15-16	Repeat meas 3-4 to change positions, girl turning under boy's Lt arm to end in Con-Pos	1-6

Second Part

Partners in Con-Pos, both facing LOD. Make progress to LOD. Boy's Lt arm extended to Lt, girl's Rt arm to Rt.

Boy's Part—Girl does Opposite

Meas		Count
1	Long step fwd on LF	1
	Swing RF fwd, toe pointed down, no wt	2-3
2	Long step fwd on RF	4
	Fwd-close L-R	5-6
3-4	Repeat meas 1-2	1-6

Repeat all to end of music in plain Waltz time. End in position to repeat 1st part.

Variation for Second Part: Partners take ClPos, boy facing LOD, girl facing opposite LOD.

Meas		Count
1-2	Waltz fwd & bwd, make ½ Lt turn	1-6
3	Waltz fwd, make ¼ Lt turn, boy facing wall	1-2-3
4	Fwd L, swd R draw L to R no wt, face LOD	4-5-6
5-8	Repeat meas 1-4	12 cts.

Use either or both variations to end of music in plain Waltz time, always ending in position to commence first part.

THE MEXICAN HOP DANCE

This is one of the simplest and liveliest of several Mexican folk numbers. Also called *La Raspa,* it is not to be confused with the far more difficult Mexican Hat Dance.

First Part

Couples form a circle, with boys facing out, girls facing in. Each start on the LF. Hands may be placed on the hips during the first 7 counts, or arms may be swung to and fro to enliven the motions.

Meas		Count
1	Hop in place on LF, push RF fwd heel down, toe up, no wt	&1-2
2	Hop and bring RF bwd to place, push LF fwd, heel down, toe up, no wt	&3-4

3	Hop and bring LF bwd to place, push RF fwd, heel down, toe up, no wt	&-5
	Hop and bring RF bwd to place, push LF fwd, heel down, toe up, no wt	&-6
4	Hop and bring LF bwd to place, push RF fwd, heel down, toe up, no wt	&-7
	Hold this position. *Clap Hands TWICE!*..	&-8
5-8	Repeat meas 1-2-3-4, starting the hop on RF	&1-&8
1-8	Repeat the entire 8 measures.........	&1-&8 &1-&8

Note that the hops are all executed on the "&" count!

Second Part

Partners face each other as at the beginning of the First Part.

MEAS		COUNT
1-4	Hook Rt elbows. Both start on LF, take 8 steps to complete a roundabout to the Rt. Release elbows, then	1- 8
5-8	Hook Lt elbows. Both start on LF, take 8 steps to complete a roundabout to the Lt. Release elbows, then	1-8
9-12	Hook Rt elbows. Both start on LF, take 8 steps to complete a roundabout to the Rt. Release elbows, then	1-8
13-16	Both move to Lt, boy hooks Lt elbow with next girl on his Lt, girl hooks Lt elbow with next boy on her Lt, then take 8 steps to complete a roundabout to the Lt.........	1-8

With new partners, repeat First Part, then Second Part. Continue to end of music.

THE HORA

The basic movements of the Hora are common to dances in several European countries, among them Greece, Yugoslavia, and Romania. The Hora, however, has become the national dance of Israel. It can be danced to several Israeli tunes, and is sometimes executed with leaps and bounds and with voices geared to the rhythm in shouts of joy and exuberance.

First Part

Partners are not necessary, just a circle of boys or girls—or boys and girls! Hands are extended along the adjoining person's arms, gripping elbows; or the hands may be extended across to opposite shoulders. Keeping in time with the music, the movements start slowly and are speeded up as the dance progresses.

1st Variation

Meas		Count
1-2	Swd on LF, then cross RF behind LF	1-2, 3-4
3	Swd on LF, HOP on LF, swing RF front	5-6
4	Step-HOP on RF to Rt side, swing LF in front	7-8
5-8	Repeat meas 1-4	1-8

2nd Variation

1-2	Swd on LF, cross RF behind LF	1-2, 3-4
3	Swd on LF, HOP on LF swing RF in front	5-6
4	Swd RF, do ball-change L-R	7&8
5-8	Repeat meas 1-4	1-8

3rd Variation

1-2	Swd-close L-R, swd-close L-R	1-2, 3-4
3	Swd LF and lean Lt, ball-change R-L	5&6
4	Swd RF and lean Rt, ball-change L-R ...	7&8
5-6	Repeat meas 1-4	1-8

4th Variation, Used to changed direction

Meas		Count
1-2	Swd LF, cross RF behind LF	1-2, 3-4
3	Swd-close L-R and twist to face Rt	5-6
4	Fwd on LF, then ball-change R-L	7&8

Note that the 4th variation is ended with weight on the LF so that the 1st, 2nd, or 3rd variations can be started on the RF. Any of the movements can be used over and over, or a set number of either in sequence used to match the phrasing of the music.

Second Part

Use the same formation as in the First Part

Meas		Count
1	Two quick steps diag fwd on L-R	1-2
2	Jump on both feet bringing them together .	3-4
3	HOP on LF, then swing RF fwd	5-6
4	Take 3 stomping steps feet together R-L-R	7&8
5-8	Repeat meas 1-4	1-8

When change of direction is desired: HOP on RF, swing LF fwd on cts. 5-6; take 3 stomping steps on L-R-L, cts. 7&8.

THE MISIRLOU

This dance had its origin in Greece. On its arrival in America it became a popular fun outlet at both private parties and in many night clubs. Its pattern is short and simple, and it can be danced to Tango rhythms. The formation can be a circle of four or more, or a single line of boys and/or girls. Partners are not necessary.

Meas		Count
1	Swd on RF to LOD, then point LF across RF	1-2
2	Twist body to Lt, cross LF in back of RF.	3
	Twist body Rt, step fwd on R-L to LOD.	&-4
	Repeat as desired	
3	Bwd-close-bwd on R-L-R	1&2
4	Fwd-close-fwd on L-R-L, end facing center	3&4

Square Dancing

Square Dancing has been in vogue since Colonial days, when it was an important part of America's social life. Get-togethers of all kinds—quilting parties, corn-husking bees, barn raisings—often wound up with a shindig at which perhaps the only rhythmic effects were the clapping of hands, stomping of feet, and singing and chanting of various rhythmic patters, the latter sometimes composed on the spot by the caller and the jubilant participants. In many instances this would be the only type of sound permitted, since a fiddle, banjo, or harmonica would have classified the activity as "dancing" which, because of religious tenets, would have been forbidden by the ministers and elders of certain sects. Square Dances were sometimes then, and even now, referred to as "Barn Dances". Many of them were actually held in barns, since few ballrooms or halls were to be found in the rural areas where these affairs had their start.

When invited to a Square (or Barn) Dance today, you should be prepared to indulge in not only those patterns and movements commonly known as Squares, but also an occasional Circle, Contra, Quadrille, and Folk Mixer; maybe a Patty Cake Polka, a Paul Jones, and a Virginia Reel. There are hundreds of Square Dance patterns and figures, all appropriately named: Chicken Reel, Chase the Rabbit, Duck for the Oyster, Hinkie Dinkie, Red River Valley, and on and on and on! All are designed to create fun and frivolity, plus plenty of physical exertion.

An important factor in Square Dancing is the ability of the leader, referred to as the "caller," to apply with perfect rhythmic incantation the "singing" and "patter" calls which provide instructions for the dancers to follow. The spirit and personality injected into these calls account for much of the vigorous response on the part of the dancers, and rattling off the patters can be compared with an auctioneer's efforts to obtain more dollars for the item up for sale.

The music for Square and Folk Dances and for Party Games and Mixers is written mainly in 2/4 time. Records for Square Dances are available with and without the directional calls.

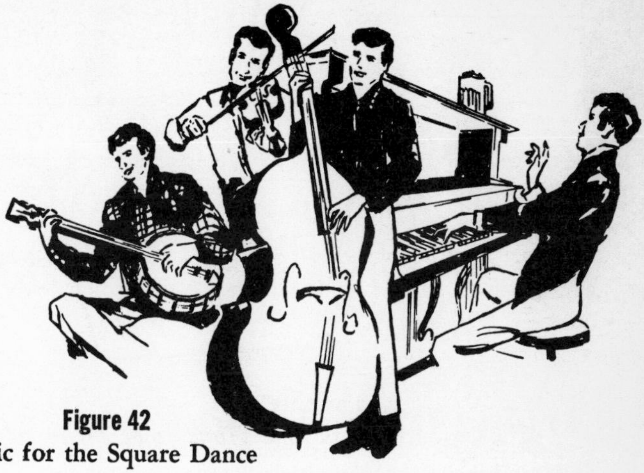

Figure 42
Music for the Square Dance

BASIC SQUARE DANCE FIGURES

All Square Dances, regardless of their name or the tune to which they are danced, consist of a predetermined sequence of basic figures and patterns. Once efficiency is attained in executing these basic movements, it should not be difficult to understand and follow the directions sung out by the caller.

The Square Set

Four couples occupy floor space of about eight to ten feet square. Numbered counterclockwise, the first or head couple stand with backs to the caller facing couple three, and two and four face each other.

The first call is usually *Honor Your Partner!* followed by *Honor Your Corner!* Partners face each other, the boy bows to the girl and the girl curtsies to the boy; they each then turn and the boy bows to the girl on his left, while the girl curtsies to the boy on her right. The music for this movement is two chords sounded by the orchestra.

Figure 43
The Square Set

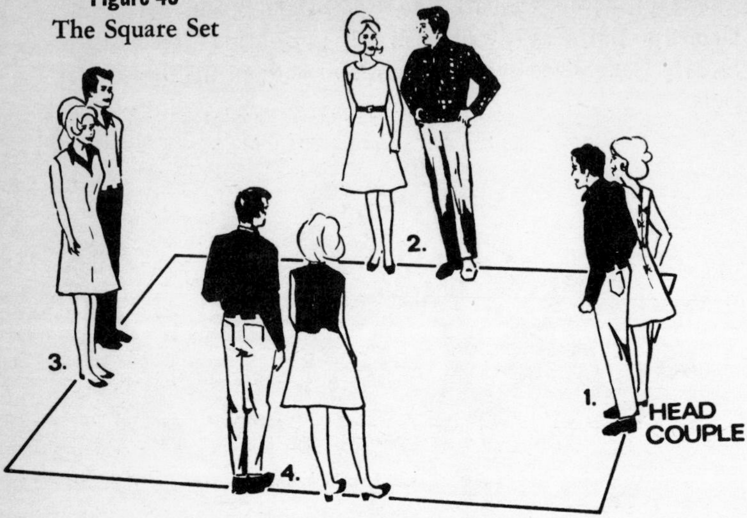

The Circle

The next call could be *All Join Hands and Circle to the Left* (opp. LOD) or Right (to LOD). A complete circle is made back to the couples' original positions. This could be done with a swd-close repeated over and over, usually with a lively hop and skip action; or it could be done with a progressive walking step (eight or sixteen counts).

The Promenade

Now the caller might sing out with a *Promenade All!* In either of the two positions shown the couples can either walk, do a step-close-step (cha-cha-cha) or a lively hop and skip (sixteen counts).

The Balance and Swing

Partners face each other, join right hands. Then both step left on LF and swing RF across in front of LF; then step right on RF and swing LF across in front of RF (eight or sixteen counts).

The Closed Swing

Partners face each other to start one of the liveliest and, for some dancers, the most difficult type of movement. The

Right Swing is most widely used. The simplest form is a full change of weight from one foot to another, with a sharp turning movement of the body. However, the dancer will eventually develop the ball-change movement, which is done by both partners placing the weight forward on the RF, then pressing the ball of the LF slightly sideward and backward (ball) to allow the Rt heel to raise and lower slightly (change), thus creating a slight pivot to the right. The movement can be applied to both the Elbow Open Swing and the ClPos Swing (eight counts).

The Elbow Open Swing

With right elbows linked this can be done with either a walking step or with the ball-change and pivot, as in the Closed Swing. The direction is clockwise. With left elbows linked and with weight for both on LF forward, a counterclockwise pivot turn can be done (eight counts for each).

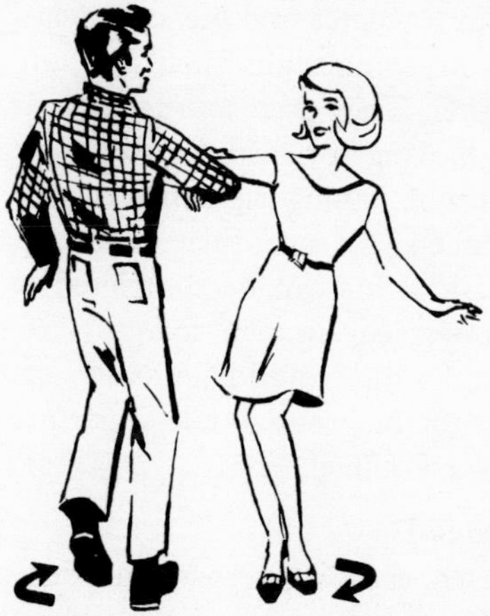

Figure 44
The Elbow Open Swing

The Allemande Left

The dancers all face their *corners!* Left hands are joined and a complete roundabout is made, counterclockwise, ending facing partners and releasing corner's hands (8 counts). This could be followed by a *Swing Your Partner!*

The Allemande Right

Partners face each other, join Rt hands, make a complete roundabout and end facing each other, with boy facing LOD, and girl the opposite (eight counts).

The Grande Allemande

The boy and girl make progress as in the Grand Right and Left: the boy toward LOD, the girl opposite LOD. To start, partners link right elbows as in the Elbow Swing and make a complete right swinging turn. Release elbows, proceed to next boy and girl, link left elbows and make another complete turn, this time to the left. Again release elbows and repeat right and left until partner is faced. As with the Grand Right and Left this figure can be done with Square Sets of four couples or with several couples in circle formation. In the latter this would be a change of partner game, with the leader signaling when to take a new partner. (Eight counts for each turn).

The Grand Right and Left

Partners face each other, join Rt hands and move forward (boy to LOD, girl opposite), brushing right shoulders and let go hands in passing each other. They then join left hands with next boy or girl and keep moving forward, brushing left shoulders, releasing left hands and joining right hands with the next and so on until they once again meet their own partners. With a speedy hop and skip this can be completed in eight counts; with a slower movement sixteen counts is required. When used in Party Games the Grand Right and Left is continued until the caller signals the group to take a partner when either right or left hands are joined.

The Do-Si-Do

Facing partners, hands released, each walks forward brushing Rt shoulders in passing. Then each moves to the right—*without turning*—and steps backward, brushing left shoulders in passing, and into original position. Two couples can do the Do-Si-Do thus: couples one and three or, couples two and four walk toward each other, brushing right shoulders with opposite boy or girl. Both couples then move sideward to right, walk backwards, brushing left shoulders with opposites and return to positions in the set (eight counts).

The Ladies' Chain

The caller signals either the head couples (one and three) or the side couples (two and four) to start this figure. The boys remain in their position while the girls walk forward, join Rt hands, brushing right shoulders in passing. As they pass they release Rt hands and give Lt hands to opposite boy. With the girl's Lt hand in his Lt hand he puts his Rt arm around her waist and does a Chain Turn, he moving backward, the girl forward. The girls now do the Chain again and return to their partners who repeat with them the Chain Turn. A total of sixteen counts is required for this figure.

The Star

This figure can be done by four boys, four girls, or two couples, depending on the caller. In some cases the entire set of four couples is called upon to do the Star. Usually started with Rt hands to the center and circling clockwise, it can be reversed by the dancers turning around and extending Lt hands to the center and circling counterclockwise.

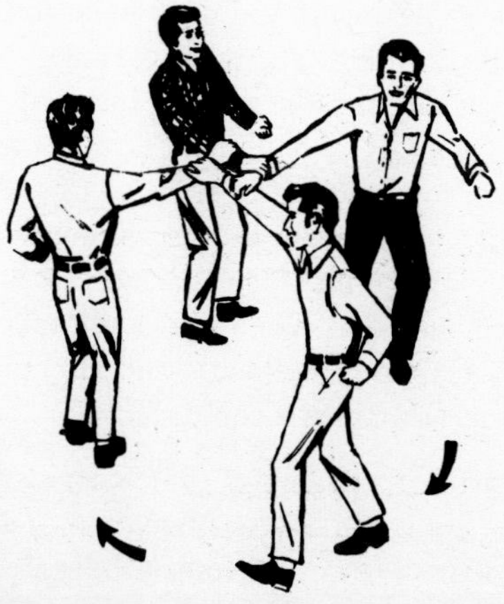

Figure 45
The Star

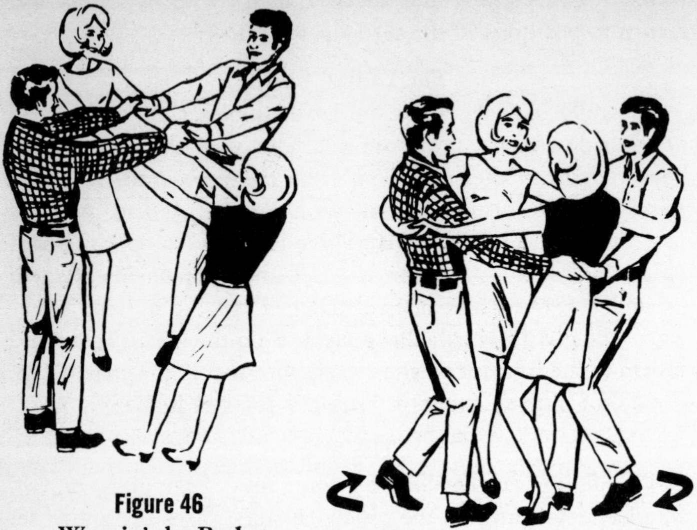

Figure 46
Weavin' the Basket

Weavin' the Basket

Head couple moves to right and joins hands with the second couple, circling left for eight counts. Releasing hands, the boys join hands with each other, the girls doing likewise with their hands clasped under the boys' hands. The boys then raise their hands, extend them past the girls' heads and drop them to the girls' waistlines. The girls do likewise, thus forming the Basket in eight counts. Then all take the weight forward on the RF, then use the LF to start a ball-change movement which develops into a Circle to the left for eight counts. All then release hands and return to places in the set, ending with a Swing Your Partner for eight counts. The Basket can then be done by the couples three and four. The couples not taking part can liven things up by clapping the hands and stomping the feet in time to the music (thirty-two counts).

Let it be understood that the foregoing is to be considered as the basic, or elementary, approach to the formation of the numerous and varied Square Dances. Group leaders and callers conceive and use additional figures and patterns; sometimes a group reaches the stage where the leader's imagination is taxed in order to keep abreast of the progress being made by the group. The music plays an important part in Square Dancing; for instance, *Turkey in the Straw* would most likely suggest a different sequence from that danced to *Nellie Bly*. There is the possibility, too, that a change of tunes will suggest vastly different rhythmic responses and physical reactions on the part of the dancers.

THE VIRGINIA REEL

This old-timer is a long time favorite, especially those who enjoy, but seldom have the opportunity to perform, Square Dancing. It is termed a Longways Dance, and is made up of the easier square dance steps and figures. Once a sequence of movements has been set, the crowd will have little difficulty in following the pattern; as a consequence, a skilled caller will not be required to sing out the directions in which the participants are to move. The formation is usually a line of boys and a line of girls facing each other, boys toward LOD, girls opposite LOD. The head couple would be at the far right, next to the wall; the foot couple at the far left, or center. Six couples make an ideal set, but more can be added if the crowd warrants.

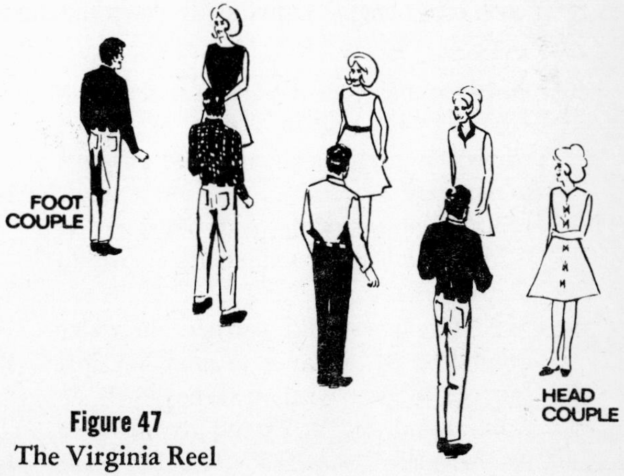

Figure 47
The Virginia Reel

The Howdy Do

MEAS		COUNT
1	Both lines 4 steps fwd, partners pat Rt palms	1-4
2	Both lines 4 steps bwd, clap hands	5-8
3	Both lines 4 steps fwd, partners pat Lt palms	1-4
4	Both lines 4 steps bwd, clap hands	5-8
5-6	Partners join Rt hands, do walk-around to Rt	1-8
7-8	Partners join Lt hands, do walk-around to Lt	1-8
9-10	Partners join both hands, walk-around to Rt	1-8
11-12	Partners DO-SI-DO	1-8
13-14	Head couple join hands, hop-skip down center	1-8
15-16	Head couple hop-skip back to place	1-8

On the walk-arounds and the DO-SI-DO, partners end in original positions.

The Reel

In this the head couple starts by reeling themselves, and then reels each other couple individually down the line, thus:

MEAS		COUNT
1-2	Head couple join Rt elbows, do walk around to Rt, release elbows, extend Lt elbows to opp lines (boy to next girl, girl to next boy)	1-8
3-4	Join Lt elbows with next boy/girl, do walk-around to Lt, extend Rt elbows to partner	1-8
5-6	Join Rt elbows with partner, do walk-around to Rt, advance to next boy/girl	1-8
7-8	Join Lt elbows with next boy/girl, do walk-around to Lt, extend Rt elbow to partner	1-8
9-10	Join Rt elbows with partner, repeat meas 5-6	1-8
11-12	Join Lt elbows with next boy/girl, repeat meas 7-8	1-8

13-14	Join Rt elbows with partner, repeat meas 9-10	1-8
15-16	Repeat meas 11-12 with next boy/girl . . .	1-8

On completion of meas 15-16 head couple prepares to head down the center to original places. During the reeling the others waiting their turn to be reeled enter into the spirit by clapping hands and/or tapping the floor with one foot.

Under The Arch

After swinging the sixth couple, the head couple proceeds down the center thus:

Meas		Count
1-2	Boy takes girl's Rt hand in his Lt, both return to places in line	1-8
3-4	Boys face to Rt, girls face to Lt (toward wall); head boy circles to Rt and leads boys' line to foot of set; head girl circles to Lt and leads girls' line to foot of set. .	1-8
5-6	(Head couple meet and form the arch: both)	1-8
7-8	(Hands raised high overhead)	1-8
7 to 16	2nd, 3rd, 4th, 5th and 6th couples now proceed under the arch, making progress toward wall to reform set. The couple forming the arch remains in place, becoming the 6th, or foot couple. The former 2nd couple is now the head couple	1 to 8

Repeat from the beginning.

CULTIVATING MUSICAL RESPONSE

A good Square Dancer should be able to apply the varied movements to the indicated number of musical beats and measures. Once the "feel" of square dance music has been absorbed the dancer will respond to its rhythmic accent and automatically move in and out of an 8-count phrase. The caller's intonation of the directives and the patters plays a large part, too. Most Square Dance figures are set to four bars of music (eight counts); among these are the Circle and the Do-Si-Do. Figures like the Grande Allemande and the Promenade take up sixteen counts.

ARRANGING A SQUARE DANCE

The orchestra, and many records, start off by sounding two introductory chords. On the first the caller will command HONOR YOUR PARTNER! On the second, HONOR YOUR CORNER! And then the fun begins. The following group of figures can be danced to any of several tunes: *Irish Washerwoman, Pop Goes the Weasel, Sugar in my Coffee-O, Buffalo Gal,* and many others.

As explained before, hundreds of varied sequences have an equal number of names, so the sequence that follows could be called, for want of a better name, *Shindiggin' at the Hoedown!*

SHINDIGGIN' AT THE HOEDOWN

A.	Honor Your Partner!	Chord
B.	Honor Your Corner!	Chord
1.	Head Couples UP and Forward & Back .	8 cts.
2.	Side Couples UP and Forward & Back .	8 cts.
3.	Head Couples UP & Do-Si-Do	8 cts.
4.	Side Couples UP & Do-Si-Do	8 cts.
5.	Allemande LEFT (Corner)	8 cts.
6.	Allemande RIGHT (Partner)	8 cts.
7.	Grand Rights & Left	8 cts.
8.	Repeat Grand Right & Left	8 cts.
9.	Ladies' Chain—1st Part	8-cts.
10.	Ladies' Chain—2nd Part	8 cts.
11.	Swing Your Partners	8 cts.
12.	Swing Your Corners	8 cts.
13-14.	Grande Allemande	16 cts.
15.	Meet Your Partner & Balance & Swing.	8 cts.
16.	Now to Your Corner & Balance & Swing	8 cts.

Weave the Basket (Couples 1 and 2)

17.	a. Join Hands & Circle Left	8 cts.
18.	b. Form the Basket	8 cts.
19.	c. Circle Left	8 cts.
20.	d. Back to Places	8 cts.

Weave the Basket (Couples 3 and 4)

21.	a. Join Hands & Circle Left	8 cts.
22.	b. Form the Basket	8 cts.

23.	c. Circle Left	8 cts.
24.	d. Back to Places	8 cts.
25.	a. Gents to the Center, Form The Right Hand Star	8 cts.
26.	b. All change Hands, Form The Left Hand Star	8 cts.
27.	c. Ladies Join Partners in The Left Hand Star	8 cts.
28.	d. Promenade All to Your Places in the Set	8 cts.
29.	Head Couples UP and Do-Si-Do	8 cts.
30.	Side Couples UP and Do-Si-Do	8 cts.
31.	All Hands UP & Circle to the Right	8 cts.
32.	All Turn around and Go the Other Way.	8 cts.

The figure sequence can be changed to suit the participating group's liking; however, a change in the lettered figure sequence might prove confusing. Note that each group of four figures is set to 32 counts, or 16 bars of music, for a total of eight 16 bar phrases. Once the timing of the figures has been accomplished the Patters can be applied to provide even more fun and frolic in Square Dancing.

APPLYING DIRECTIONAL AND PATTER CALLS

A successful Square Dance caller should be able to convey to the dancers the figures and patterns used in the proper sequence and also to inject singsong patters, many of them made up on the spot. Three types of patters have been developed and used the country over:

The Introduction Patter, used to liven up the action of getting the crowd onto their feet and into the sets.

The Break, Swing, and Promenade Patters, used in changing from one pattern to another, and to liven up the action.

The Closing Patter, used in shooing the crowd off the floor and to the refreshment tables at the end of a number.

In setting the count for the patters, the accent is always on the word or syllable corresponding to the numerical expression. Each is based on four bars of music.

Introductions

TIGHTEN up your BELT and BUTTON up your VEST
1 & 2 & 3 & 4
Get UP and grab the GAL you THINK is BEST
& 5 & 6 & 7 & 8

GRAB that BABE and PAT HER on the CHEEK
1 & 2 & 3 & 4
And if SHE socks YOU go JUMP in the CREEK
& 5 & 6 & 7 & 8

INTO your PLACES and ON with the BALL
1 & 2 & 3 & 4
TIGHTEN up your BRITCHES for a GOOD long HAUL
5 & 6 & 7 & 8

Breaks, Swings, Promenades

You WHIS – tle FIRST and THEN you SING
& 1 & 2 & 3 & 4
Then you ALL join HANDS and FORM a big RING
& 5 & 6 & 7 & 8

ALL join HANDS in a GREAT big RING
1 & 2 & 3 & 4
Now MAKE your FEET go BING bing BING
& 5 & 6 & 7 & 8

SWING your GAL and then OH by HECK
1 & 2 & 3 & 4
DON'T you DARE do a DIS – co – TEK
5 & 6 & 7 & 8

SWING her HIGH then SWING her LOW
1 & 2 & 3 & 4
Then SQUEEZE her TILL she HOL – lers WHOA
& 5 & 6 & 7 & 8

SWING your GAL as MUCH as you PLEASE
1 & 2 & 3 & 4
Let the OTHER guy LOOK at her DIM – pled KNEES
& 5 & 6 & 7 & 8

SWING her DOWN and SWING her UP
1 & 2 & 3 & 4
SWING her HARD and YELL hup HUP
5 & 6 & 7 & 8

SWING the GAL who LOVES you BEST
1 & 2 & 3 & 4
Then TIGHTEN your BELT and HEAD out WEST
& 5 & 6 & 7 & 8

GRAB that GAL in CAL – i – co
1 & 2 & 3 & 4
LET her KNOW you're ON the GO
5 & 6 & 7 & 8

Closing Patters

Get OFF the FLOOR and ALL head SOUTH
& 1 & 2 & 3 & 4
And TAKE a bit of MOON – shine IN – to your MOUTH
& 5 & 6 & 7 & 8

GRAB your GAL and TAKE her off the FLOOR
1 & 2 & 3 & 4
I'LL YELL when it's TIME to come BACK for MORE
& 5 & 6 & 7 & 8

That's ALL there Is there AIN'T no MORE
& 1 & 2 & 3 & 4
WALK your PART – ners OFF the FLOOR
5 & 6 & 7 & 8

TAKE your GAL to a ROCK – in CHAIR
1 & 2 & 3 & 4
FOR THAT'S the END of THIS ole SQUARE
& 5 & 6 & 7 & 8

OLD king COLE and his FIDD – lers THREE
1 & 2 & 3 & 4
Can't PLAY no MORE till they've HAD a little SPREE
& 5 & 6 & 7 & 8

Party Games and Mixers

REGULARLY scheduled social dance activities conducted by schools, churches, YM-YWCA's, etc., use games and mixers to keep the wallflowers from blooming too profusely, and to give the bashful boys and girls a chance to get an occasional partner without asking. Sometimes the group leader is a dance teacher who has taught the group a number of "fun dances"; in any event, usually someone is present who can "call" a Paul Jones or Circle Dance to help keep the crowd on the move.

A well-organized group will have on hand several records to which games can be danced; perhaps the orchestra, if one is used, can play old-time tunes like *Turkey in the Straw, Virginia Reel,* etc. Some of the simpler and equally effective games can be danced to any lively Fox-Trot or Polka. The only other properties necessary to conduct a round of mixers are (1) a whistle, one used by coaches and referees, and (2) a sharp, clear voice which carries well and which can, when necessary, make the calls in sing-song with the music being played.

Often referred to as "ice-breakers," these mixers are popular with all age groups. Anyone with a good sense of timing and a flair for projecting personality can easily become a "mixer-upper." Group leaders attest to the fact that a two-fold purpose is served by using mixers: they provide fun for the crowd and, best of all, new acquaintances are made without formal introductions.

THE DOUBLE CIRCLE

This is one of the more widely used ice-breakers, one that will get all hands off their chairs! With music playing, lower the volume, then:

1. Give a sharp toot on the whistle to attract attention. Invite all the dancers and sitters to *form two circles* . . . girls on the OUTSIDE, face in . . . boys on the INSIDE, face out.

2. When the circles are formed call: ALL JOIN HANDS AND CIRCLE TO THE RIGHT! Both circles move in opposite directions.

3. With circles in motion, blow whistle and call: GRAB THE ONE NEAREST TO YOU AND DANCE!

4. Allow crowd to dance with this partner for about 30 seconds, then call again for the circles to form. This time it could be with boys in the outer circle, girls in the inner circle.

THE MULTIPLICATION DANCE

This is another easy game for the group leader to start in motion. One couple is selected to start: it could be the tallest boy and the shortest girl, or the boy in the blue suit and the girl in the pink dress. Then proceed as follows:

1. The music starts and the couple selected begins to dance. The group leader asks those on the sidelines to *give the starting couple a hand!*

2. After a few seconds of dancing, the whistle is blown and the dancing couple separates to choose other partners.

3. At short intervals, signal the dancing couples to separate and take other partners—*always the nearest person from among those not yet dancing.*

4. With the entire assembly on the floor, the stage is set for a follow-up with any one of several other mixers.

THE LEMON DANCE

This is a "mixer" which is extremely popular with younger dancers—from the fourth through the seventh grades. It serves as a good follow-up for the Multiplication Dance.

Depending upon the size of the group, select one or more couples. Give each boy and girl a lemon; each of them uses the lemon to "tag" another boy or girl and dances with the partner of the person who was given the lemon. The one who now has the lemon gives it to someone else, and so on.

The game continues at the discretion of the leader; five to eight minutes is suggested. The music is stopped suddenly—in the middle of a bar—and the whistle is blown. Those caught with the lemon in hand stand on chairs or a platform and *eat the lemons*—without sugar, of course!

SELECTING LEAD-OFF COUPLE FOR MARCH ON REFRESHMENTS

After an hour of instruction and dancing, a sixth grade class can develop a terrific hunger and thirst. The well-intended announcement that "refreshments are served" can produce good-natured bedlam plus an overturned table or two.

A fun game to use in this situation is to select the *last couple to be served.* It prevents the usual chaos, and the "winning" couple seldom if ever objects to the honor bestowed—especially if an extra soda or ice cream is offered as a prize!

1. Form a circle of couples, with girls at boys' right, all facing LOD. Space the couples two to four feet apart.
2. Explain the rules: the winning couple will bring up the rear of the line of couples marching to the refreshment tables.
3. Group leader, standing in center of circle, promises to keep both eyes shut as he makes several fast pivots to right and left.

4. Completing the turns, he stops suddenly and, with both eyes still covered, points to the lucky pair!
5. The march to the refreshment tables is started, with the couple that was behind the winning couple leading the line.

THE POLKA'S PART IN FUN DANCING

With its springy, bouncy rhythm, the Polka has always been a dance for fun and frivolity. Several years ago there was devised one of the many versions of the Polka suited to those lacking the ability or the desire to exert themselves with the "hop, skip, and jump" necessary in the Round or Standard Polka. It called for a succession of progressive steps, with no turning, toward LOD. Called the "Jessie Polka," it was basically a fun dance. The tune best suited for this dance was, strangely enough, a recording by a Dixieland Jazz Band, the *A & E Rag*!

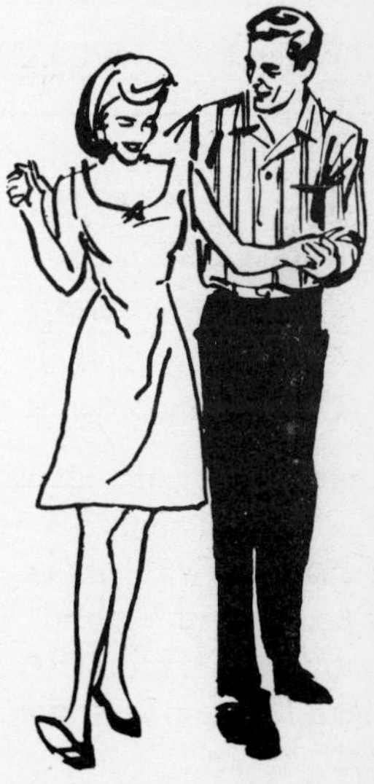

Figure 48
The Cowboy Cha-Cha

Members of the Young Adult Dance Club of the Central Queens (New York) YMCA, supervised for many years by the author, adopted the Jessie Polka as their very own, and during the heyday of the Cha-Cha in the late 1950's they nicknamed this dance the "Cowboy Cha-Cha."

The Cowboy Cha-Cha

The Square Dance version of Prom-Pos is used throughout: facing LOD, lady at man's right side, his right arm circling her waist, his right hand clasping her right hand. His left and her left hands are clasped in front, shoulder high. Progress is toward LOD. Both start on left foot and do the same steps.

Start feet together:	COUNT
Extend LF fwd, heel down, toe up	1
Close L to R............................	2
Extend RF bwd, toe down, heel up..........	3
Touch R at side of L.....................	4
Extend RF fwd, heel down, toe up..........	5
Close R to L............................	6
Extend LF fwd, heel down, toe up..........	7
Touch L toe at right side of RF...........	8
Cha-cha-cha fwd L-R-L..................	1-&-2
Cha-cha-cha fwd R-L-R..................	3-&-4
Cha-cha-cha fwd L-R-L..................	5-&-6
Cha-cha-cha fwd R-L-R..................	7-&-8

Summarized, the above can easily be remembered: counts 1-2 on LF; counts 3-4-5-6 on RF; counts 7-8 on LF; then cha-cha-cha fwd 4 times.

Once the timing and steps have been developed, try this: lean bwd on 1, straighten on 2; lean fwd on 3, straighten on 4; lean bwd on 5, straighten on 6; lean bwd on 7, straighten on 8.

The Patty Cake Polka

Here is another fun dance in the Polka family which is a favorite with all ages, since it does not require the overly strenuous efforts needed in some of the other Polkas. It is done in a circle of couples, or two circles if the size of the crowd wàrrants. Partners face each other, boys with backs to the center, girls with backs to the wall. Little or no progress is made either toward or opposite LOD. To start, both hands are joined and raised outward.

First Part

Boys Part–Girls do Opposite

MEAS		COUNT
1	Swing LF swd, heel down, toe up, no wt ..	1
	Point Lt toe in front of Rt toe	2
2	Repeat cts. 1-2	3-4
3	Swd-close L-R and repeat	5&6&
4	Swd-close L-R, then swd-draw L-R	7&8&
5	Swing RF swd, heel down, toe up, no wt ..	1
	Point Rt toe in front of Lt toe	2
6	Repeat cts. 1-2	3-4
7	Swd-close R-L and repeat	5&6&
8	Swd-close R-L, then swd-draw R	7&8&

Variation: As the Swing and Point is made on the LF and RF (counts one to four) hop slightly on the other foot simultaneously with the Swing and Point. Also, boys' hands can be placed at the girls' waists and girls' hands on the boys' shoulders.

Second Part

MEAS		COUNT
1	With Lt palm boy pats her Rt palm 3 times.	1&2
2	With Rt palm he pats her Lt palm 3 times .	3&4
3	With both palms he pats her palms 3 times ..	5&6
4	Both bend, pat own knees 3 times	7&8
5-8	Hook Rt elbows and with 4 *cha-cha-cha's* .	1&2 3&4
	make complete roundabout, release elbows	5&6 7&8

Repeat 1st and 2nd parts to end of music.

Variation: On signal from group leader, or on instructions at the start, on releasing elbows at end of turn boys may move on to the next girl on their left, and the girls to the next boy on their left, thus effecting a change of partners.